PRINCIPLES OF LOWER-EXTREMITY BRACING

Edited by
JACQUELIN PERRY, M.D., and
HELEN J. HISLOP, Ph.D.

Published by
AMERICAN PHYSICAL THERAPY ASSOCIATION
1156 15th Street, N.W. Suite 500
Washington, D.C. 20005

Copyright 1967
by the American Physical Therapy Association

Second Printing—1970

Third Printing—1972

Fourth Printing—1973

Fifth Printing—1977

Sixth Printing—1978

Seventh Printing—1980

Library of Congress Card Catalog Number: 67-31337

ISBN 0-912452-16-1

Preface

THE STAFF of the Rancho Los Amigos Hospital, Downey, California, was invited by the American Physical Therapy Association to present Instructional Courses on the Principles of Lower-Extremity Bracing at its Annual Conferences in 1966 and 1967. This monograph is an outgrowth of those sessions. The articles appeared in the September 1967 issue of *Physical Therapy,* Journal of the American Physical Therapy Association.

Rancho Los Amigos Hospital has received international acclaim for its contributions to orthotics and to the concepts of rehabilitation of patients with long-term or chronic disease.

The hospital is unique in that the size of its clinical program has permitted disability groups commonly found in rehabilitation centers to be separated into special treatment units of fifty to sixty beds each. There are services for spine and hip deformities, spinal cord injury, stroke, fractures and amputations, arthritis, cerebral palsy, and for chronic chest disorders as well as a cardiac rehabilitation service. As a result of this type of organization, the staff has been able to concentrate much more thoroughly and intensively on the specifics of each disability.

They have demonstrated that there are basic principles of function and orthotic management common to all patients, but that optimum success with rehabilitation rests with recognition of the unique problems of each type of disability and modification of the principles and techniques appropriately. The organization of this monograph reflects their experience.

Reproduction of normal walking mechanics is the goal of treatment, regardless of type of disability. But the exact manner of replacement of lost function varies quite markedly. Thus the chapter designations include disability groups such as: "Structural Insufficiencies," "Control Dysfunction," and "Flaccid Paralysis."

Determination of the best approach to bracing requires pooling of the specialized knowledge and experience of the different members of the therapeutic team. The background of the physician best fits him to identify the patient's disability, his total needs, and the related pathomechanics. The physical therapist's background and detailed contact with the patient give him the opportunity to analyze the patient's performance, and initiate appropriate recommendations for a functional program. The orthotist, with his colleagues in engineering, is best equipped to determine how the patient's functional needs will be translated into steel, leather, or plastic.

This monograph reflects the philosophy at Rancho Los Amigos, that close integration of clinical management, research, and education is essential for optimum patient rehabilitation. Treatment inadequacies are identified through patient service and solved through research. Inclusion of the research advances into the clinical program is accomplished through education.

Students in any of the health professions will find value in this monograph—either for detailed instruction in the principles of lower-extremity bracing, or for overview of the bracing needs for specific types of patients.

Physical therapists, physicians, and orthotists in practice will particularly find this monograph helpful in their day-to-day management of the patient with severe disability. The depth and breadth of knowledge presented is unique in this subject area.

Hopefully the authors will expand their writing at a future time to include upper-extremity, trunk, and neck bracing.

HELEN HISLOP, PH.D.
Editor, Physical Therapy
American Physical Therapy Association
New York, New York
December 1967

Contents

Introduction 7

THE MECHANICS OF WALKING: A Clinical Interpretation—*Jacquelin Perry, M.D.* 9

Relationship Between Lesion Specificity and Bracing—*Jacquelin Perry*, M.D. 33

PARALYTIC DYSFUNCTION

    I. Pathomechanics—*Jacquelin Perry*, M.D. 36

    II. Bracing the Unstable Knee in Flaccid Paralysis—*Marilyn J. Lister*, B.S. 38

    III. Brace Design for Flaccid Paralysis—*David Heizer*, C.O. 48

    IV. Bracing for Patients with Traumatic Paraplegia—*Elwin Edberg*, B.S. . 50

    V. Long-Leg Brace Design for Traumatic Paraplegia—*David Heizer*, C.O. 56

CONTROL DYSFUNCTION

    I. Pathomechanics—*Jacquelin Perry*, M.D. 59

    II. Control of Lower-Extremity Movement in Cerebral Palsy—*Virginia Scaramuzza Guess*, B.S. 63

    III. Bracing the Unstable Knee and Ankle in Hemiplegia—*Margaret Inaba*, B.S. 70

    IV. Short-Leg Brace Design for Hemiplegia—*David Heizer*, C.O. 76

STRUCTURAL INSUFFICIENCY

    I. Pathomechanics—*Jacquelin Perry*, M.D. 81

    II. Structural Insufficiencies of the Knee in Rheumatoid Arthritis—*Virginia Scaramuzza Guess*, B.S. 86

    III. Bracing Design for Knee Joint Instability—*David Heizer*, C.O. 92

Introduction

LOWER-EXTREMITY BRACING must meet the dual requirements of adequate stability for standing with sufficient flexibility to step ahead so as to provide optimum assistance for walking. Attention to the requirement of mobility is a fairly new approach in orthotics and the designs presented in this monograph cannot be considered final. Rather they are the devices the staff at Rancho Los Amigos Hospital has found most effective to date. We expect many of the techniques of bracing presented in these pages to undergo modification and refinement as our knowledge of the biomechanics of walking becomes more sophisticated.

No attempt has been made to present the history of the development of the various brace designs because so little of this information has been recorded in the literature. The functional long-leg brace is an excellent example: it evolved directly from advances in the field of prosthetics. The first applications of the principles of the quadrilateral socket to orthotics were made by Bidwell in Milwaukee and Scott in Denver. At the time these men made this breakthrough, their attention was diverted to more pressing matters because the need for these braces waned with the rapid eradication of epidemic poliomyelitis. Thus their experience with functional bracing was never published for others to share.

Undoubtedly original contributions to brace design have been made in other localities with equal lack of publication of experience or results. As a consequence, we have been able to give recognition only to those published references and to those persons with whom we have had personal exchange of information and ideas.

Readers should consider this monograph to be an interim report of lower-extremity bracing. The brace designs and the criteria for application have been used successfully in patient management and thus they constitute our clinical recommendations to date. However, the fluid state of the art and science of orthotics and the current surge for better educational and research programs strongly indicate major advances to be made in the next few years.

For these reasons, the principal emphasis in the Instructional Courses from which this monograph was derived was on pathomechanics and the clinical interpretation of walking patterns. Familiarity with such basic knowledge, combined with one's own clinical observations and the contributions of modern technology, will be the basis of future bracing designs which will replace the best we have to offer today.

The goal of bracing is to meet the functional requirements of a disabled patient while offering him minimal restriction.

We hope that the reader will derive two sources of stimulation from these pages: (1) new methods of brace application which will improve patient management, and (2) the urge to seek additional refinements in brace design through the application of space-age technology to the solution of problems of human motion today.

JACQUELIN PERRY, M.D.
Rancho Los Amigos Hospital
Downey, California
December 1967

THE MECHANICS OF WALKING

A Clinical Interpretation

JACQUELIN PERRY, M.D.

WALKING IS FREQUENTLY described as a simple act of falling forward and catching oneself. If this is so, why does the person who has recovered some 50 to 60 degrees of knee flexion and has good quadriceps strength, still limp following casting for a fractured femur? Why does the hemiplegic patient walk poorly when he can flex and extend his paretic extremity quite well? Answers to these kinds of questions have stimulated numerous persons throughout the past century to investigate the actual mechanics of walking.

Improved instrumentation and close teamwork between medicine and engineering permitted Inman, Eberhart and their associates [1,2,3] to define and expand the works of earlier investigators.[4,5,6] As a result, they have provided temporal and qualitative relationships, as well as more explicitly delineated, the fundamental components of walking. These components are the arcs of joint motions, sequence of muscle actions, and rates of body advancement, trunk alignment and ground force reactions.

Subsequent to these studies valuable additions, confirmations and refinements have been contributed independently by Murray [7,8] and Sutherland.[9] The efforts of these many investigators have clearly identified the complex mechanics of walking. Modern prosthetic practice depends heavily on these data, and some of the information has been applied to tendon transplant surgery,[10] but little if any of the data have been incorporated in the management of the many other disabilities which constitute the bulk of orthopedic practice. This omission appears to result from fragmentary publication, presentation of data in obscure reports, and adherence to unfamiliar terminology and strange frames of reference. Scientific investigators find significance in value changes of each variable independently, whereas the clinician attributes significance only to those factors which demonstrably influence the patient's ability to perform. This is not to say that one is more important than the other, but to note the way different persons use data. For the clinician to utilize the scientist's findings, the data must be reinterpreted into functional terminology and concepts.

Reinterpretation of the data on walking is the purpose of this paper.

FUNCTIONAL TASKS OF WALKING

Though sometimes used for recreation, walking is basically a means of travel from one place to another—a way of reaching a position to see, to hear, to perform a manual task. Therefore, walking is of secondary importance and should require only minimal amounts of time and energy. In addition, the body needs a smooth ride so as to avoid jarring the sensitive tissues that comprise the brain, the heart and other vital organs, if top performance is to be retained. Smoothness and energy economy are best accomplished by a wheel traveling over an even surface.[3] But wide variations in both natural and man-made terrain are everyday experiences. These obstacles are better handled by the versatility of multijointed limbs.

To closely approximate the smoothness and energy economy of a wheel, and yet retain the ability to accommodate irregular terrain, man's two lower extremities pass through an intricate series of muscle and joint actions. During the course of travel three functional tasks are accomplished: (1) forward progression, (2) alternately balancing the body over one limb and then the other, and (3) repeated adjustment of relative limb length. Each has its own mechanical demands and responses (Table 1).

Forward Progression

The multitude of actions related to advancing the body in a smooth and economical manner may be grouped into three functions: absorption of the shock related to a rapid transfer of weight on to the forward foot; control of momentum that threatens the stability of the limb as a weight-bearing structure; and, generation of sufficient force to carry the body forward. By clever utilization of momentum to assist in shock absorption and in propelling the

```
TABLE 1
FUNCTIONAL TASKS OF WALKING
Forward Progression
    Shock Absorption
    Momentum Control
    Forward Propulsion
Single Limb Balance
Limb Length Adjustment
```

body forward, the work requirements are minimized in all three of these tasks. The details of these accomplishments will be discussed as the total walking cycle is analyzed.

Single Limb Balance

To advance by the use of two limbs, the individual must be able to balance the body over one limb while swinging the other. Without such balance (or an adequate substitute) he cannot walk.

When standing in the traditional erect posture, the trunk is well centered between the two supporting limbs. As soon as one foot is lifted to take a step the body becomes grossly off-balance because of the loss of one of these supports (Fig. 1A). The person would fall unless (1) there is a massive holding force from the hip abductor muscles, and (2) he shifts laterally over the weight-bearing foot. Both actions are utilized in normal walking.

The normal person shifts his weight prior to attempting to take a step. In fact, he appears incapable of lifting his foot without this shift. Persons with normal proprioception and muscle control, but who lack adequate hip abductor stability, either because of paralysis of the abductor muscles or mechanical inefficiency at the hip joint (from old fractures or dislocations), substitute by exaggerating the lateral shift of the trunk (Fig. 1B). Patients who are not capable of sensing this need to shift weight, such as the hemiplegic patient with limited proprioception and disturbed central control, will fail to substitute. This will cause him to fall toward the unsupported side as the foot is lifted (Fig. 1C).

The normal individual walks with his feet about 3 inches apart.[7] He thus needs to move over only an inch to realize an effective compromise of muscle action and alignment stability (Fig. 1A). This seems very minor, but with the body weight locking the foot on the ground

A CLINICAL INTERPRETATION

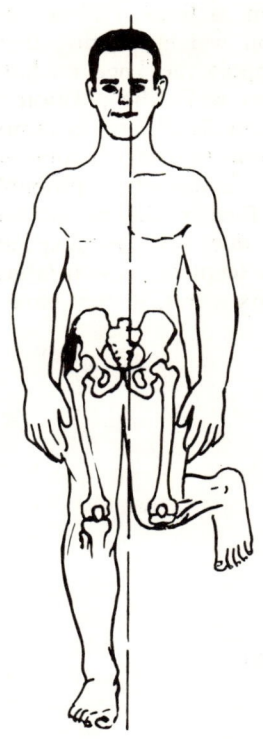
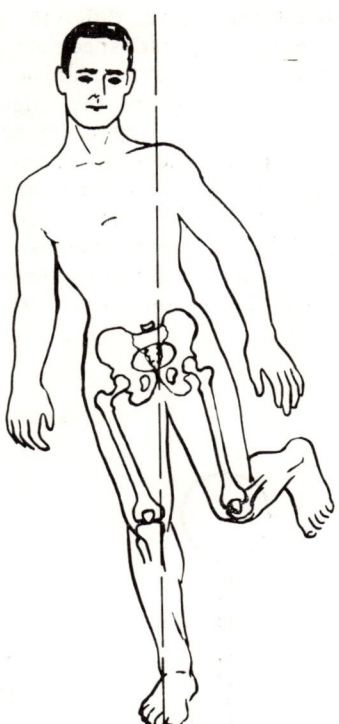
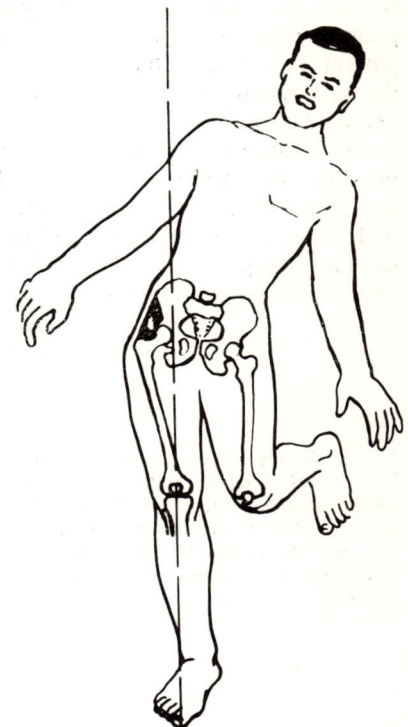

STANDING
NORMAL STANCE HIP ABDUCTORS
STRONGLY ACTIVE

A.

STABLE
POSTURAL SUBSTITUTION FOR
PARALYZED HIP ABDUCTORS

B.

UNSTABLE STANCE
INACTIVE HIP ABDUCTORS
NO POSTURAL SUBSTITUTE

C.

FIG. 1A. The normal individual balances on one limb by shifting his weight slightly to that side (approximately one inch) and by holding forcefully with the hip abductor muscles.

FIG. 1B. A person with intact sensation but an inadequate abductor mechanism (such as a poliomyelitis patient with paralysis of the gluteus medius-minimus complex) balances on one limb by shifting the trunk laterally in order to substitute trunk weight for the absent abductor force.

FIG. 1C. When a person has inadequate proprioception or body image to substitute for non-functioning hip abductor muscles he will be unable to balance on one limb. Instead he will fall toward the unsupported side (a positive Trendelenberg test).

there is a significant lateral thrust (valgus thrust) on the knee and foot (Fig. 2). This seems to account for the valgus knee deformities which occur so readily in patients with rheumatoid arthritis and those paralyzed from poliomyelitis. Experience with the paralytic patient has taught that ligaments deprived of the protection of muscular action yield to repeated strain.

The anatomy of the knee indicates two possible mechanisms to protect the ligaments by controlling the valgus thrust associated with single limb balance (Fig. 3). Three muscles wrap around the medial side of the knee: the semitendinosus, the gracilis and the sartorius. They all have the common function of knee flexion and medial support. One is a hip extensor, one a hip adductor and the third a hip flexor. These three muscles also have different rotation actions. Thus one could speculate that on weight bearing there is a mechanism to support the knee medially against the valgus thrust while the position of the hip is changing from flexion to extension and from internal rotation to external rotation. The second protective mechanism is probably the vastus medialis. Recent studies indicate that the vastus medialis does not have a special role in knee extension except to prevent lateral dislocation of the patella. But, it may have a

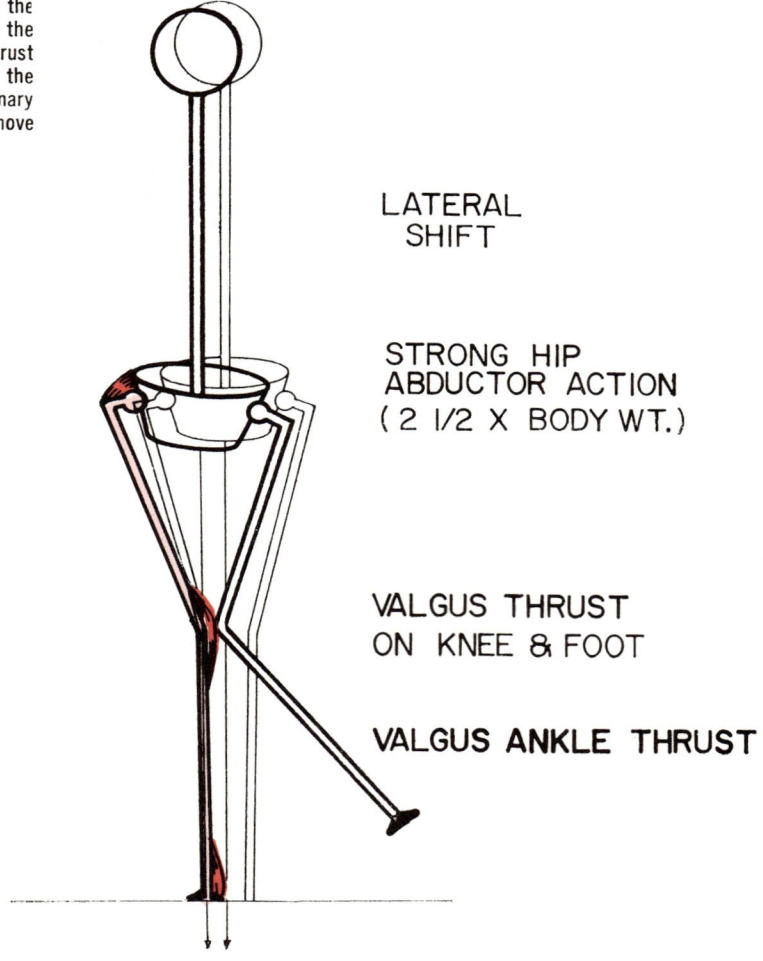

FIG. 2. As the stance phase begins the body weight is rapidly shifted toward the weight accepting foot. The major thrust of this shift occurs at the knee as the foot and leg remain relatively stationary while the trunk, pelvis and thigh move laterally.

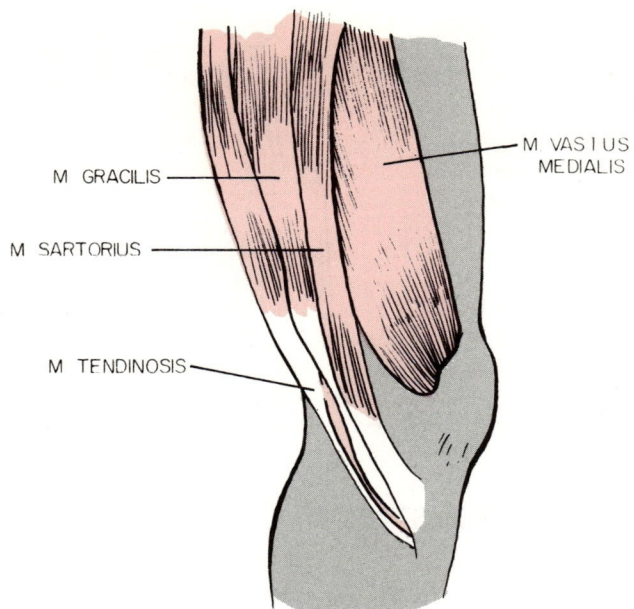

FIG. 3. The four muscles illustrated wrap around the medial side of the knee joint. Since all are active at the beginning of stance it appears that they are actively protecting the medial ligaments from the valgus thrust on the knee that occurs during single limb balance.

very important function in controlling the valgus angulation of the knee as body weight is shifted onto one foot.

A similar valgus stress occurs at the foot. The posterior tibialis muscle which becomes active as soon as weight is borne on the heel, appears to provide protective restraint. Experience with the hemiplegic patient has shown that the medial insertion of the soleus also gives some inversion, and this muscle also comes into play during the first part of weight bearing.

Limb Length Adjustment

Relative lengthening and shortening of the limb is required as the position changes to enable the foot to reach the ground with ease, whether the extremity is directed straight downward, or reaching either forward or backward (Fig. 4). Obviously, the diagonal distance between the trunk and the ground is greater than the vertical distance, and thus, the extremity which is reaching forward to take a step must be longer than the other limb which is providing vertical support. To just drop down as the body passes onto the forward foot is potentially detrimental, as evidenced by the discomfort accompanying such a jarring action. It is also inefficient, as this would cause an abrupt change in direction and hence loss of momentum that otherwise might be utilized for forward travel.

The forward reaching extremity is relatively lengthened by borrowing some of the width of the pelvis through rotating the pelvis forward with the reaching limb, and also by allowing the pelvis to drop on that side. Further length is gained from the heel by holding the foot at a right angle. Finally, the total need for length is decreased by slightly flexing the weight bearing knee.

Stress on the Hip

These motions, which accompany the swinging limb, are also creating significant stress on the hip of the stance limb. While bearing the full weight of the body plus the compressive force of the stabilizing abductor and extensor muscles, the hip passes through adduction and internal rotation and swings from flexion to extension—good reason, indeed for even minor discrepancies in the ball and socket contour of the hip joint to cause pain. These multiple stresses also mean that limitations in joint rotation will cause painful tension on the capsule and ligaments, even though the ranges of flexion and extension are still good.

Clinical experience suggests that these stresses can become symptomatic even without roentgenographic evidence of bony change.

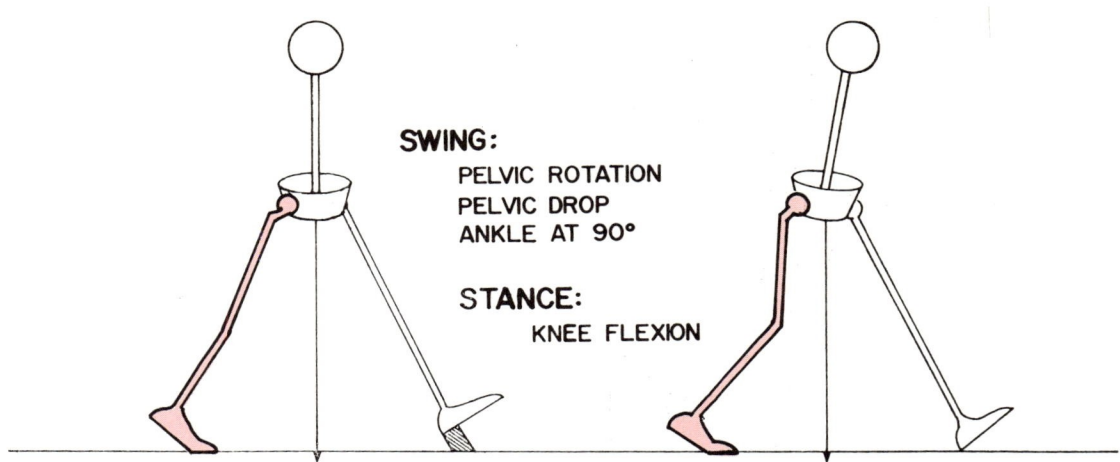

LIMB LENGTH ADJUSTMENT

FIG. 4. To reach the desired point of ground contact without dropping abruptly, the reaching limb is lengthened relatively by pelvic rotation, pelvic drop and by holding the ankle at a right angle. The demand is lessened by slight **flexion of** the stance limb.

Thus the early treatment for such disability is a program to restore the normal ranges of rotation, abduction, and extension. Obviously, painful soft tissues cannot tolerate vigorous challenge, so the exercise program must be gentle and of brief duration. The basic rule to be followed is that if the exercise causes pain, exercise, per se, is not contraindicated, but the amount of exercise has been excessive, or the method inappropriate. A person cannot walk unless he can move the limb. Hence, an appropriately graduated exercise program to improve movement is essential.

Stress on the Knee

During rotation at the hip, comparable rotatory forces are active on the knee. The stress will strain the ligaments if there is insufficient muscular strength to protect them. In addition, the person stands with the knee flexed approximately 10 or 15 degrees while he is bearing his full body weight. As a result, support is gained through muscular action rather than ligamentous tension. The quadriceps, which grasps three-fourths of the knee joint through its retinaculae, has a very vital role at this time.

THE PHASES OF GAIT

The alternate standing and stepping aspects of walking are technically defined as the *stance* and *swing* phases of gait respectively. Stance begins at "heel-strike" and ends at "toe-off." The limb then swings forward to the next heel-strike. As a means of better identifying related actions, stance has been divided into the periods of heel-strike, mid-stance, and push-off (Fig. 5). Thus the term heel-strike has been given two meanings. It may denote the initial moment of contact between the foot and the ground, or it may refer to the sequel of events resulting from ground contact. The swing phase is often divided into early and late periods.

Each of these intervals contains a complex of activity related to accomplishing a particular task. The nature of these tasks is best identified by the use of functional terminology. Appropriate functional descriptions are: weight acceptance, trunk glide, push, and balance-assist for the stance phase; pick-up and reach during the swing phase (Fig. 5). Each task is a composite of the appropriate components of forward progression, single limb balance and limb length adjustment.

A CLINICAL INTERPRETATION

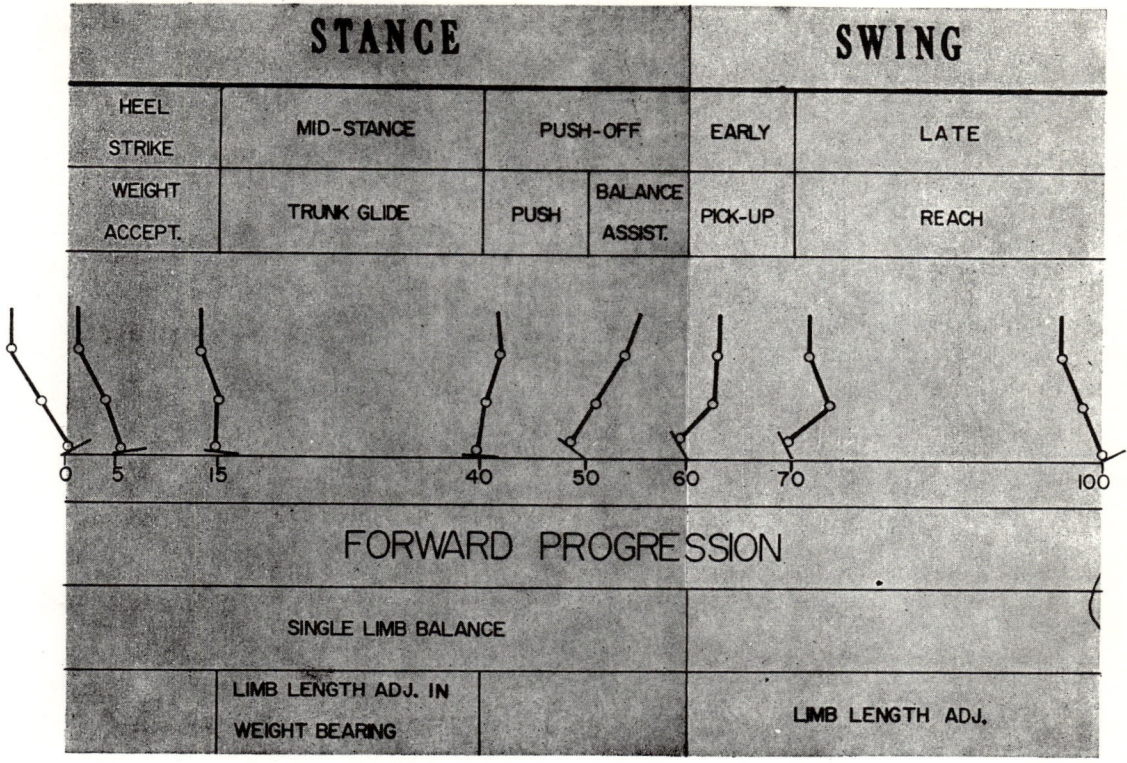

FIG. 5. The relationship between the three basic patterns of action (forward progression, single limb balance and limb length adjustment) and the subdivisions of the walking cycle are presented diagramatically. The subdivisions of the walking cycle have been identified both by time intervals (heel strike, midstance, and so forth) and by the task to be accomplished (weight acceptance, trunk glide, and so forth).

Weight Acceptance

Heel strike represents a moment of great change in demands (Plate 1). Just before the heel touches the ground, the limb was swinging forward quite rapidly as a result of its previous push-off and the active flexion at the hip and knee. To reach its forward position in time, the limb has to travel at approximately five miles an hour. At the same time the body has also received a recent forward push from the other foot so that its traveling speed is about two miles an hour. Consequently, there is considerable forward momentum in effect at the time the heel strikes the ground. Ground contact causes the foot to stop its forward travel abruptly while momentum is still tending to carry the tibia forward. If uncontrolled, this would cause the knee to collapse and the limb would be unable to support weight at the same time weight is being rapidly shifted forward and laterally from the other limb. As a result, the functional demand in the post-heel strike period is effective weight acceptance without impeding forward travel.

When the heel strikes the ground the extremity is stretched forward with the hip flexed approximately 30 degrees, the knee fully extended and the ankle is at a right angle. The weight is transmitted to the ground through the tibia, but the point of contact is at the heel, which is approximately one-third of the foot length behind the axis of the tibia. Through the leverage of this heel length, a downward thrust is created that would cause the foot to slap if it were not controlled. Control is by a rapid response of the ankle dorsiflexors (anterior tibialis and the toe extensors). Their action allows the forefoot to touch the ground gradually without a slap.

At the same time, momentum is carrying the tibia forward so that a rocker motion re-

THE MECHANICS OF WALKING

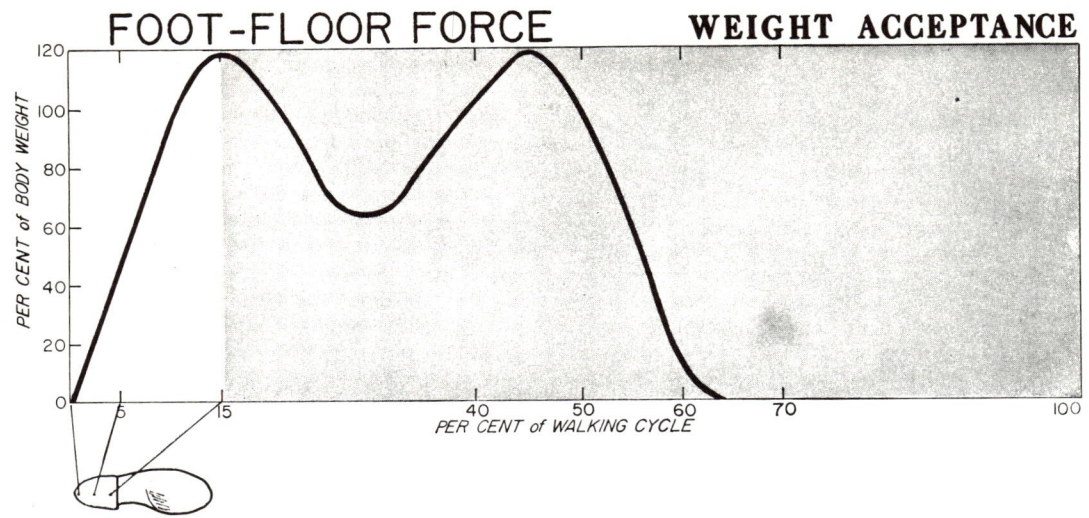

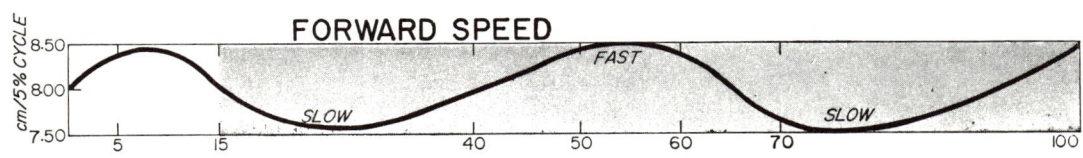

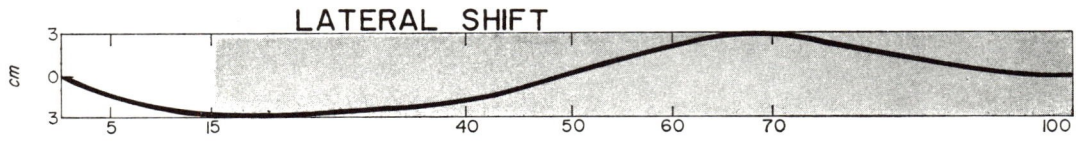

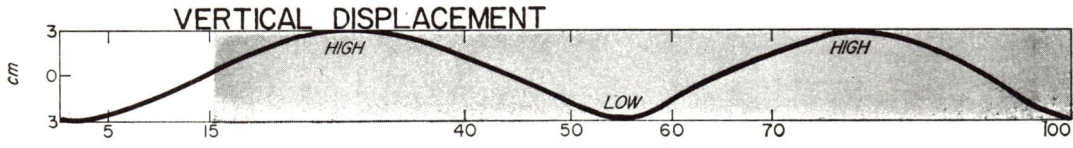

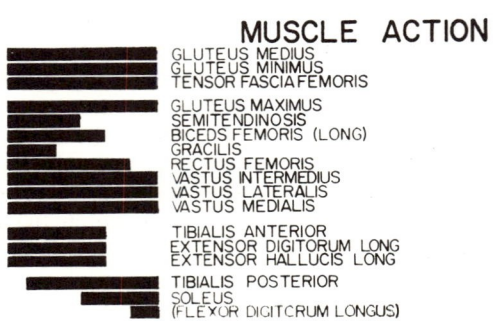

Plate 1. WEIGHT ACCEPTANCE

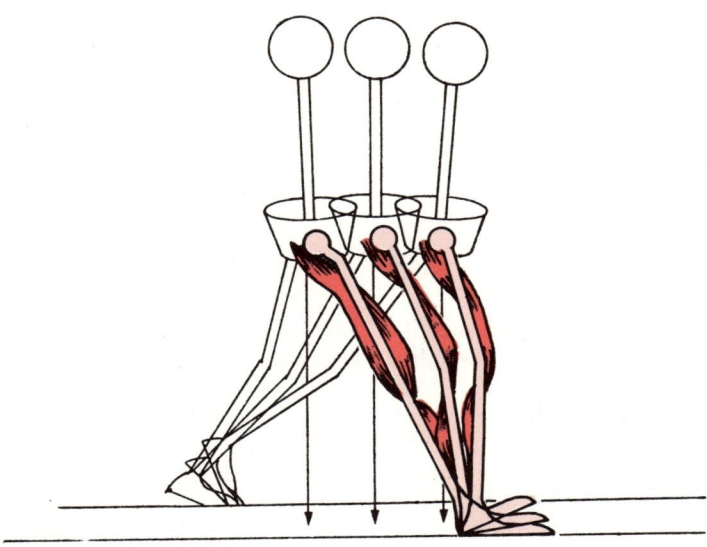

TASK: WEIGHT ACCEPTANCE (INTERVAL: HEEL–STRIKE)
Heel–Strike to Foot–Flat: 0 to 15% of Walking Cycle.

DEMANDS:
1. Shock absorption
2. Limb stabilization
3. Forward travel without interruption
4. Balance on one limb

SITUATION:
1. Strong forward momentum just before heel strike
   a. Body traveling 2 mph (force from push of opposite limb)
   b. Swing limb traveling 5 mph (force from own push plus active hip and knee flexion)
2. Extremity reaching ahead of body
3. Heel strike abruptly stops forward travel of foot; momentum now concentrated on lower leg (tibia)

RESPONSE:

Events | **Anatomical Activity**

FORWARD PROGRESSION

1. Immediate plantar flexion (due to ground contact of heel, body weight along tibia).
2. Rapid knee flexion to 15° (due to tibial advancement with thigh and trunk aligned behind foot).

3. Hip flexion tendency (due to body weight being behind weight bearing foot).

1. Restraint by ankle dorsiflexors: anterior tibialis, great and common toe extensors.
2. Knee flexion restrained by:
   a. Tibial advancement restrained by soleus and posterior tibialis
   b. Quadriceps activity
   c. Thigh stabilization through hip extensor activity by semitendinosis, biceps (long head), gluteus maximus.
3. Reversed by hip extensors and forward momentum.

SINGLE LIMB BALANCE:

1. Tendency to fall away from support limb.

2. Valgus thrust on knee secondary to lateral shift.

3. Valgus thrust on ankle.

1. Lateral shift of body. Pelvis stabilization by hip abductors: Gluteus medius, gluteus minimus, tensor fascia femoris.
2. Restrained by medial knee muscles: vastus medialis, semitendinosis, gracilis.
3. Restrained by posterior tibialis and medial insertion of soleus.

sults which allows total forward progression without any abrupt changes in direction. If this early and rapid forward travel of the tibia were not restrained, however, it would advance to a point where the extremity would become unstable because of excessive knee flexion. This is avoided by prompt action of the soleus and posterior tibial muscles which create a relative plantar flexing force. Under such control the tibia advances gradually and in a manner consistent with the dual demands of forward progression and extremity stability. Direct restraint of knee flexion is also gained by action of the quadriceps.

During this entire period of weight acceptance the body weight is still behind the weight-bearing foot and the hip is in flexion. This is an unstable position, for without control the body weight would tend to force the hip into further flexion. Action by the "hamstrings" and the gluteus maximus restrains the tendency toward hip flexion and leads to gradual hip extension.

Immediately following heel strike, two actions are occurring in the line of forward travel. One is rapid plantar flexion of the foot which is controlled by the ankle dorsiflexors. The other is rapid tibial advancement causing knee flexion, which is controlled by the soleus and posterior tibial, acting at the ankle to restrain the tibia while the quadriceps acts directly on the knee to give it support. Hip extension is also essential to control the trunk-thigh relationships. If the ankle is stabilized so the tibia cannot fall forward and the hip is prevented from flexing further, momentum will carry the thigh–body segment forward and extend the knee. Thus while the quadriceps is a very normal and useful component, it is not essential if the patient can maintain a continuous flow in his walking so as to have the assistance of momentum, in addition to tibial stability.

In addition to the forward progression challenges to weight acceptance that are occurring, demands for single limb balance also arise (Fig. 2). The latter necessitates a rapid shift laterally and a strong response from the abductor muscles.

It also means protecting the knee and ankle from the valgus thrust.

As a result of the dual demands of forward progression and single limb balance, the customary data charts indicate activity in most of the muscles of the lower extremity within the short period following heel strike.[9,11]

The data on joint motion [7] indicate increasing hip extension, increasing knee flexion and quick ankle plantar flexion followed by gradual dorsiflexion. The force charts [12] show very rapid transfer of weight onto the stance foot so that 95 per cent of the weight has been transferred within the first 10 per cent of the walking cycle (approximately 0.1 sec.). All of the work of extremity stabilization and smooth weight transfer is accomplished by the 15 per cent mark.

Trunk Glide

Following the great challenge of weight acceptance, there is a quiet period of coasting forward over the flat foot (Plate 2). Extremity stability and balance having been attained in the first period, little active effort is required now. Momentum appears to be the main propelling force as the body glides forward. In the course of this travel body weight changes its alignment from behind the heel to over the forefoot. To attain this position with minimal expenditure of energy, tibial advancement is rigorously controlled by the continued action of the soleus and posterior tibialis muscles. This allows momentum to decrease the demands of the hip and knee so that the hip muscles drop out very quickly. The quadriceps become inactive by the time the thigh has reached the vertical position, and the ankle is in about 10 degrees of dorsiflexion by the time the weight is aligned over the forefoot.

Throughout this period the body is still balanced over one leg. Hence, the hip abductors are still very active. The lateral shift, however, diminishes during the latter part of the interval as the body prepares to approach the other limb. In addition to sustained abduction stability, there is progressive internal rotation (recovery from external rotation) as the pelvis swings forward with the other limb. This accounts for the strong action of the tensor fascia femoris. This gliding period might be considered as a rest between intervals of intense work. It accounts for 25 per cent of the walking cycle, or almost half of the stance phase.

The clinical significance of this period is the need for a range of dorsiflexion at the ankle. If the tibia will not advance about 10 degrees in front of the vertical position the person loses the stabilizing effect of momentum at the hip and knee (Fig. 6A). To stand erect his knee must go into a considerable degree of hyperextension (Fig. 6B). If this is not possible, his only other means of remaining upright is to lean forward at the hips—a posture that requires good strength of the hip extensor muscles or good arm supoprt (Fig. 6C).

Push

At the end of the gliding period the body weight is in front of the foot, the knee is extended, and the heel is just rising to support the ankle against the dorsiflexing influence of the body weight that is so far forward (Plate 3). The foot is also preparing to push the body forward again. The rest of the plantar flexors become active. The gastrocnemius, the peroneals and toe flexors join the posterior tibialis and the soleus which continue their activity. The flexion action of the gastrocnemius on the knee is controlled by the forward position of body weight. Being anterior to the foot, it locks the knee in extension (there is no quadriceps activity at this time). As a result, all gastrocnemius action is at the ankle.

The combined push of the seven plantar flexor muscles creates a ground force that exceeds body weight by about 20 per cent. The speed of forward progression is increased and one might say the patient is propelled forward by the plantar flexors pushing against the ground. In the meantime the other extremity has come forward to catch the body weight as it advances. Clinically this means that the plantar flexion force is extremely important for smooth and efficient gait. This also means that the body weight is far in front of the foot and if the person lacks plantar flexion stability he cannot come up on his forefoot. He has lost a component of relative lengthening of his extremity and will accommodate by dropping the hip on that side (the so-called flat-footed gait).

During this period of marked activity at the ankle, hip control has been minimal. By having the body weight forward of the extremity

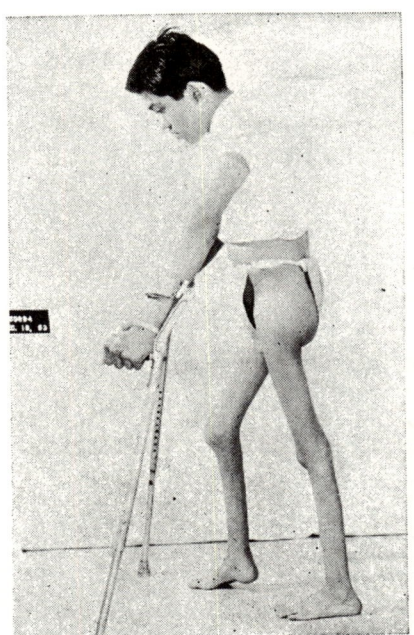
A.

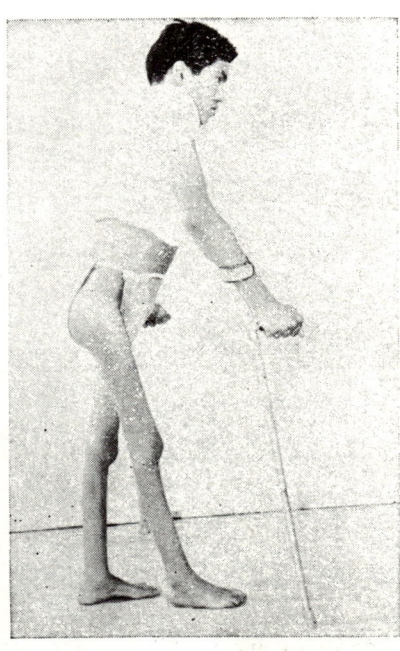
B.

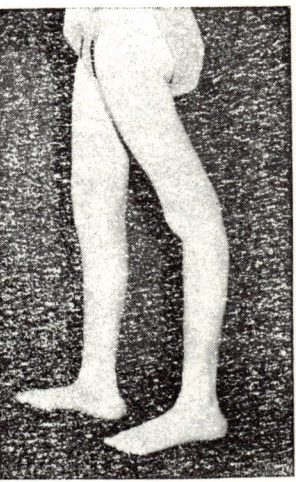
C.

FIG. 6. The patient in A and B has complete paralysis of both lower extremities resulting from poliomyelitis. He has bilateral ankle (pantalar) fusions. The left foot in A (the posterior foot in the photo) was stabilized in 10 degrees of dorsiflexion. This allows him to balance his weight over the forefoot with the hip and knee extended. Minimal crutch support is needed and no deformities have developed. In contrast, the right foot in B was fused in the traditional position of 15 degrees equinus. To bring his trunk forward over the foot on weight bearing requires considerable hip flexion. Lacking hip extensor muscles requires him to put all his weight on his arms. The relative lengthening of the right limb combined with his inability to support weight on it has encouraged hip and knee flexion deformities which add further to his instability. Fig. 6C: Lack of ankle dorsiflexion leads to exaggerated knee hyperextension as the body weight is brought forward to the weight-bearing foot.

THE MECHANICS OF WALKING

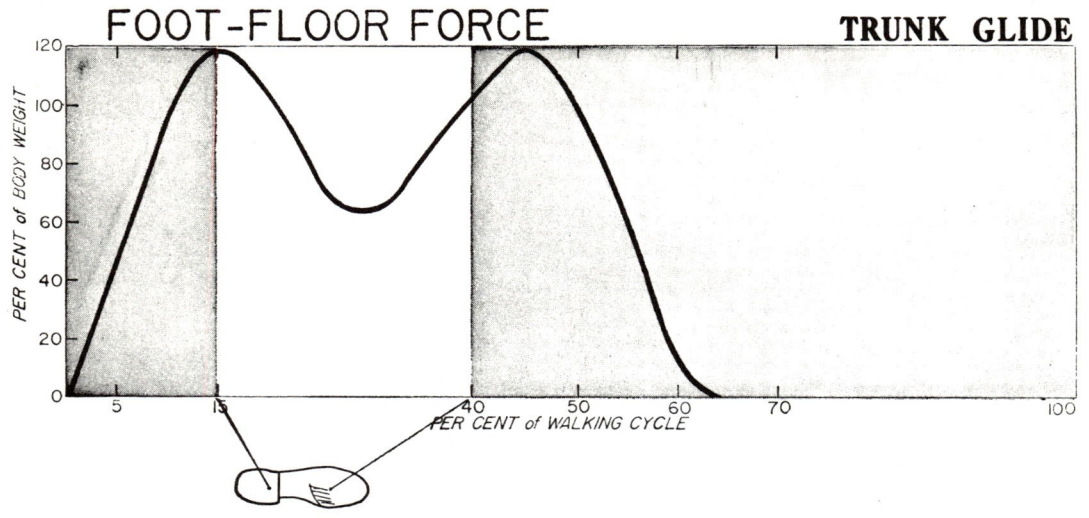

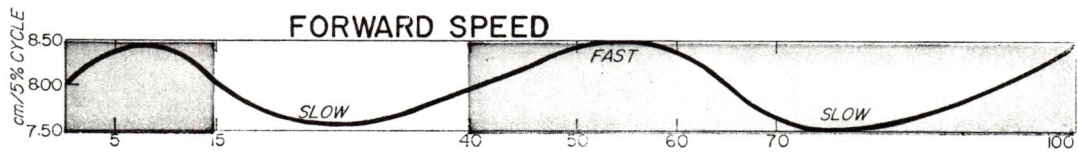

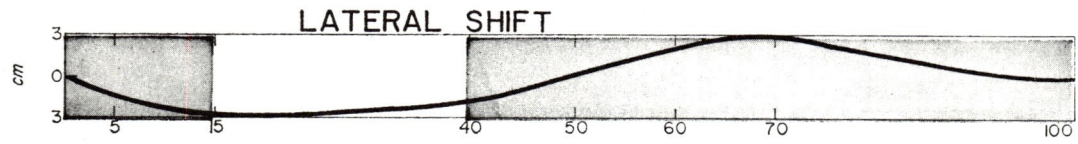

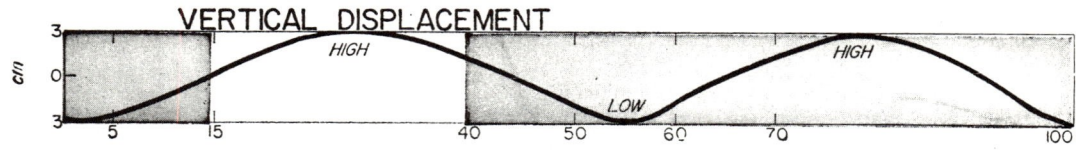

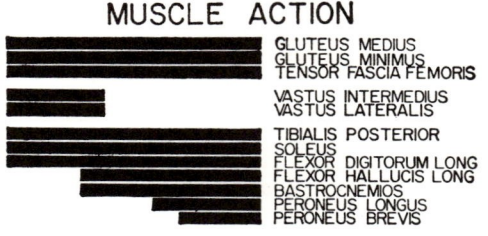

A CLINICAL INTERPRETATION

Plate 2. TRUNK GLIDE

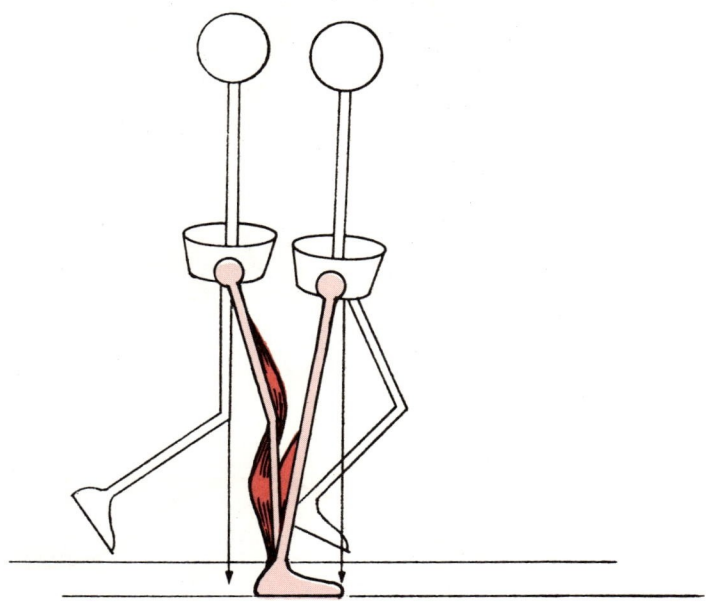

TASK: TRUNK GLIDE (INTERVAL: MID-STANCE)
Foot–Flat Period to Maximum Dorsiflexion: 15 to 40% of Walking Cycle

DEMAND:
Continue forward travel of body over flat foot.

SITUATION:
Complete single limb support has been attained.
Foot flat on the ground.
Extremity stable.
Momentum still active but lessening.
Rate of forward travel slowing a bit.

RESPONSE:

Events	Anatomical Activity

FORWARD PROGRESSION

1. Momentum carries trunk and limb segments forward over stationary foot.
   a) Knee extended as thigh advancement over stable tibia.
   b) Hip extended by thigh advancement.
2. Body weight passes from behind heel to over forefoot.

1. Rate of advancement controlled by tibial restraint: soleus and posterior tibialis activity.
   a) Quadriceps quiet.
   b) Hip extensors quiet.
2. Ankle advances from 5 degrees plantar flexion to 10 degrees dorsiflexion.

SINGLE LIMB BALANCE:

1. Total single limb support.
2. Lateral shift maximum at 20% point, then starts to decrease.

1. Continued hip abductor activity.
2. Knee stress relieved and protector muscles relaxed.

LIMB LENGTH ADJUSTMENT:
Other limb swinging forward.

Simultaneous abduction, internal rotation, and extension demand on weight-bearing hip joint.

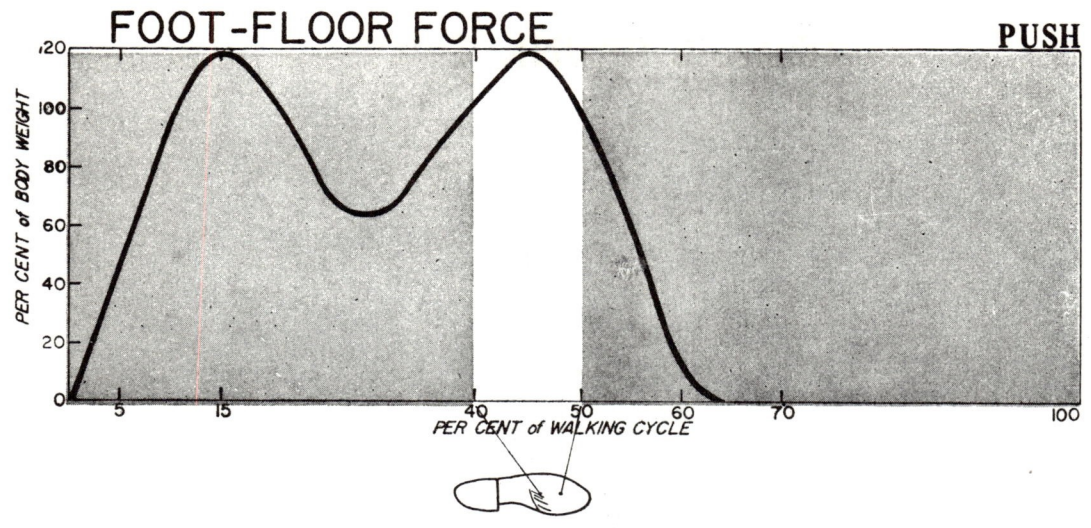
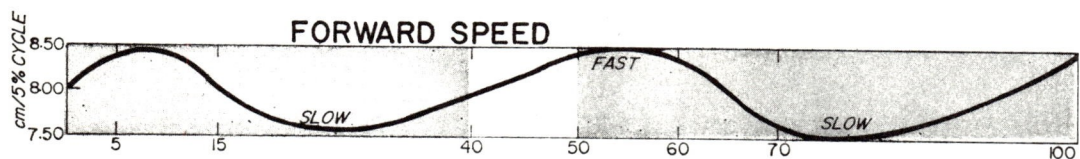
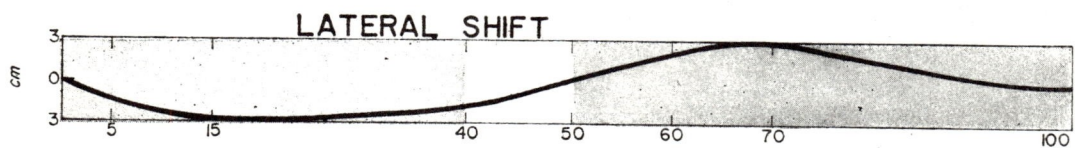
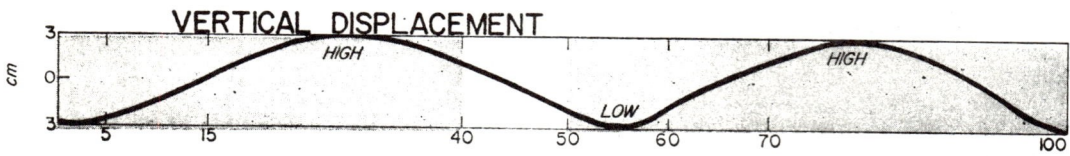
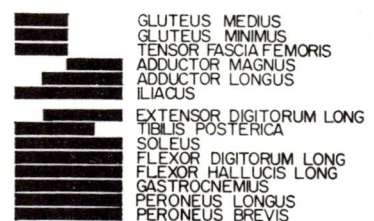

A CLINICAL INTERPRETATION

Plate 3. PUSH

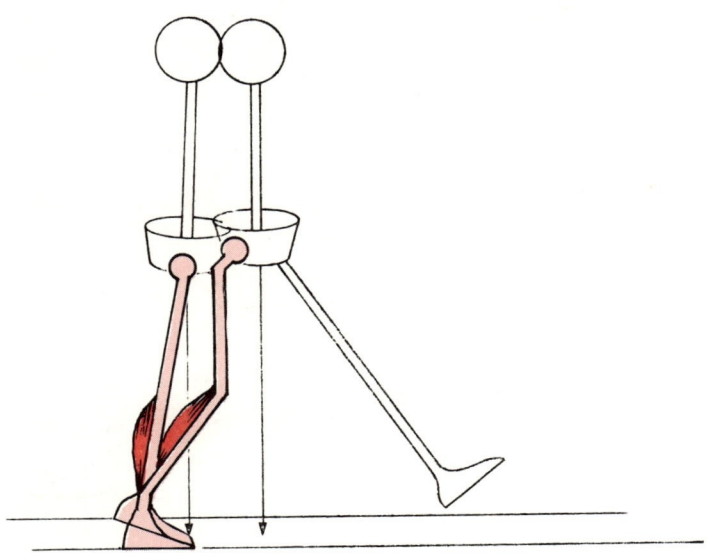

TASK: PUSH (INTERVAL: FIRST HALF OF PUSH–OFF)
   Heel–Rise to Maximum Push Force: 40 to 50% of Walking Cycle

DEMAND:
   Renew forward propelling force.

SITUATION:
   Body slightly ahead of foot.
   Knee fully extended.
   Heel just starting to rise.
   Ankle in 10 degrees dorsiflexion.

RESPONSE:

Events	Anatomical Activity

FORWARD PROGRESSION
1. Body weight tends to pull:
   a. Hip into more extension
   b. Knee into more extension
 	
   c. Ankle into more dorsiflexion
 	
2. Create push force.
	1. a. Hip extension restrained by iliacus.
	   b. Knee extension restrained by gastrocnemius to 10 degrees flexion.
	   c. All seven plantar flexors active: gastrocnemius, peroneus longus and brevis, great and common long toe flexors join soleus, and posterior tibialis which continue activity.
	2. Increased activity of all seven plantar flexor muscles.

SINGLE LIMB BALANCE: 1. Trunk returns to midline in preparation for weight transfer to other limb. 2. This creates passive abduction of hip.	1. Hip abductors relaxed by middle of period. 2. Shift controlled by hip adductors longus and magnus.

24   THE MECHANICS OF WALKING

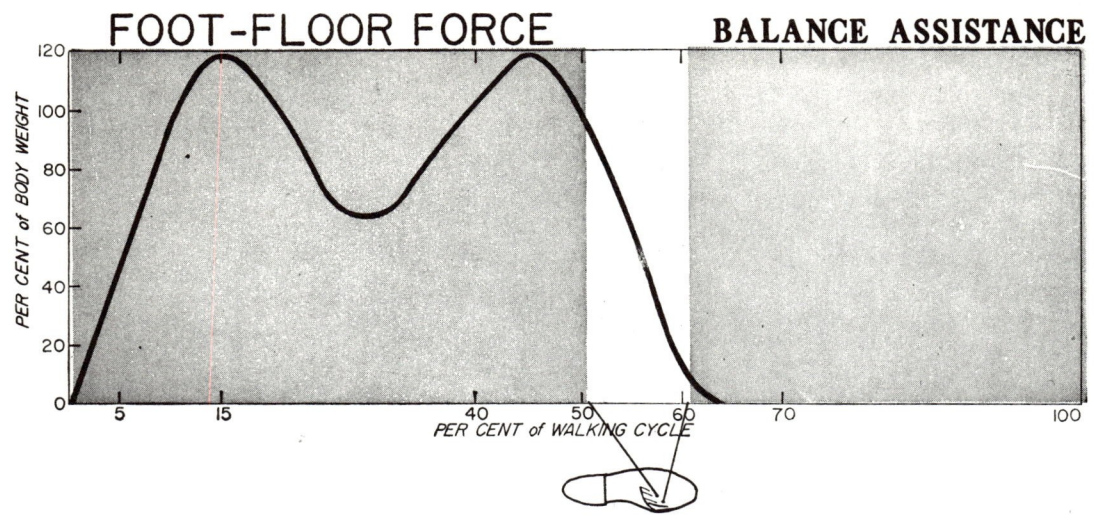

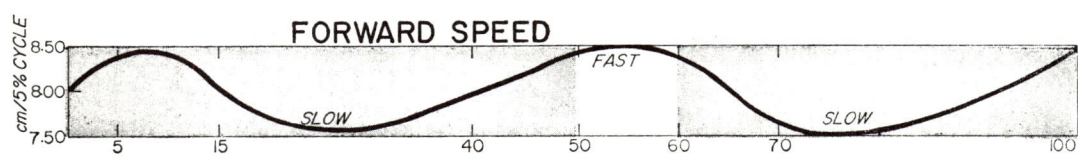

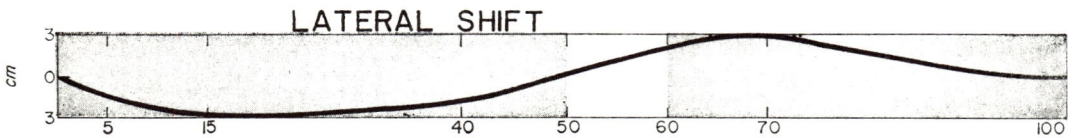

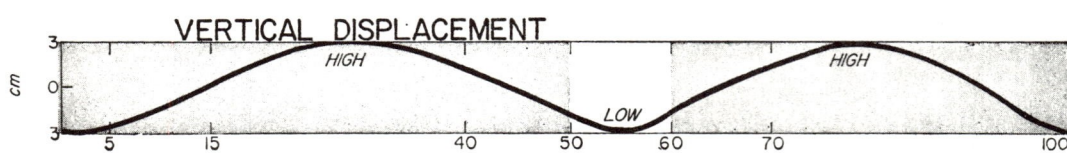

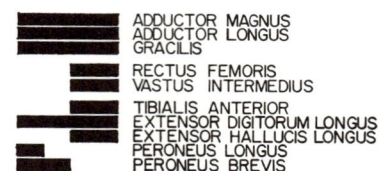

A CLINICAL INTERPRETATION   25

Plate 4. BALANCE ASSISTANCE

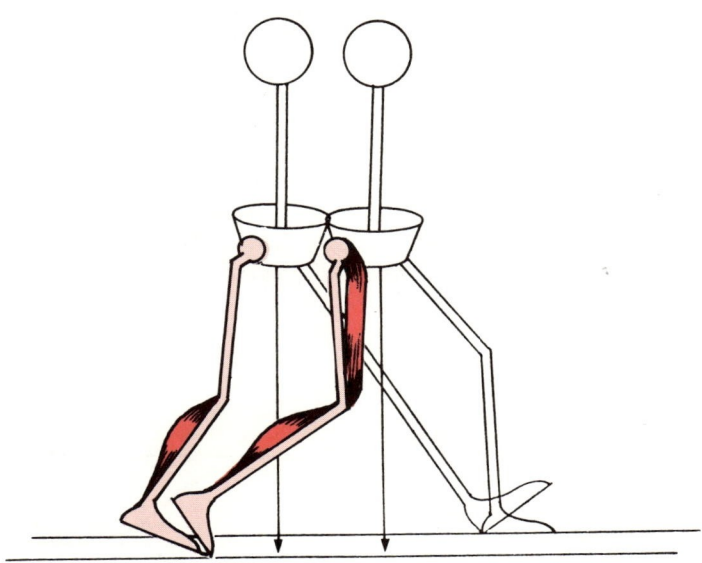

TASK: BALANCE–ASSIST (INTERVAL: LAST HALF OF PUSH–OFF)
Maximum Push Force to Toe–Off: 50 to 60% of Walking Cycle

DEMAND:
Assist body balance as other limb "struggles" to accept weight.

SITUATION:
Period of double limb support.
Weight rapidly transferred to other limb.
Primary limb maintains floor contact for balance while it prepares for swing.
Body well ahead of limb.

RESPONSE:

Events

FORWARD PROGRESSION:
1. Rapid weight transfer removes resistance at knee and ankle.
2. Floor contact maintained.

Anatomical Activity

1. Rapid and marked passive knee flexion (0 to 50°). No knee flexor muscle activity evident.
2. a. Postural equinus due to forward tipping of tibia by the knee flexion with the hip extended.
   b. Active plantar flexion: only gastrocnemius and posterior tibialis silent.
3. Hip extension lessens (−10° to 0°). Adductor longus and magnus active (let's not quibble whether this is hip joint or pelvis motion).

SINGLE LIMB BALANCE (lateral alignment)
Period of double limb support.
Weight shifting rapidly across midline to other foot.

Adductors (magnus and longus) restrain lateral shift, hence add stability.

THE MECHANICS OF WALKING

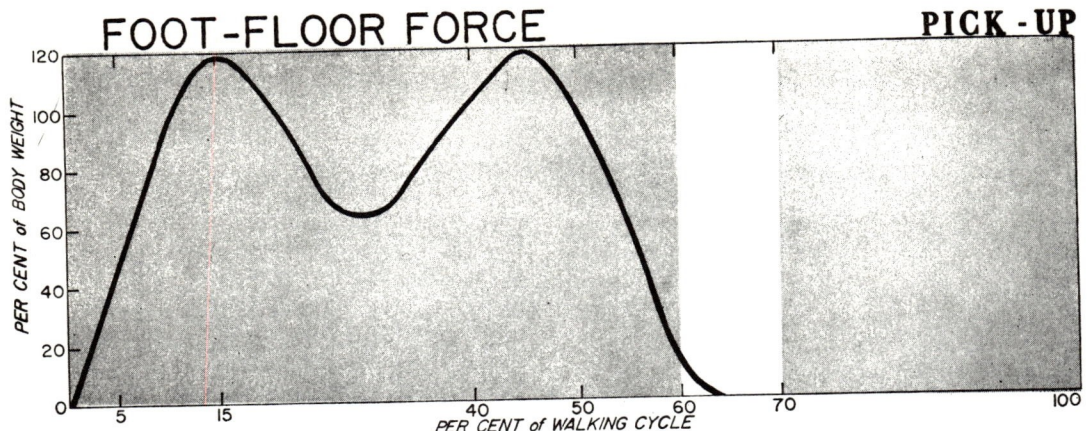

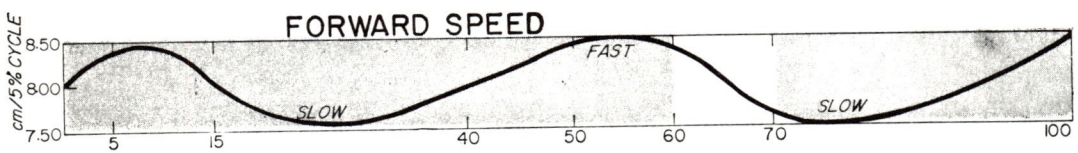

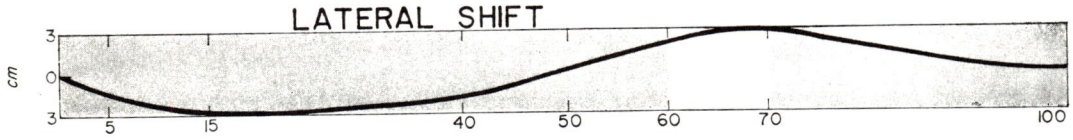

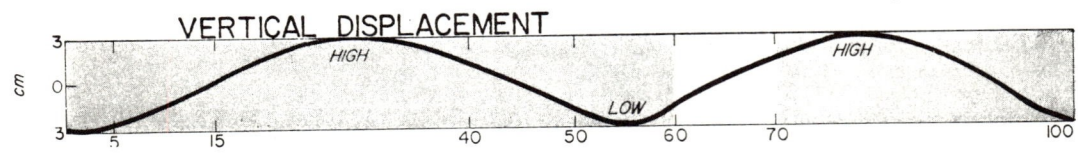

MUSCLE ACTION

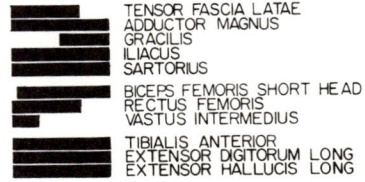

A CLINICAL INTERPRETATION

Plate 5. PICK-UP

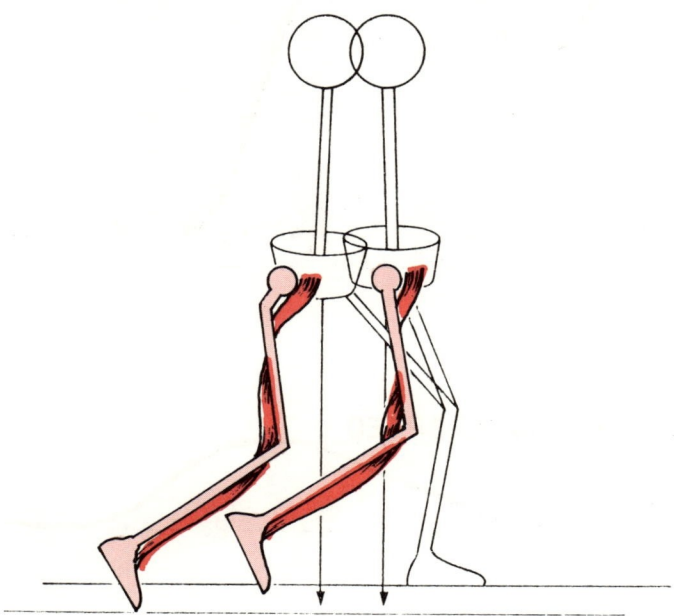

TASK: PICK–UP (INTERVAL: EARLY SWING)
Toe–Off to End of Knee Flexion: 60 to 75% of Walking Cycle

DEMAND:
   Lift foot from ground in preparation for forward reach.

SITUATION:
   Weight entirely on other limb
   Extremity far behind body axis
   Toe extended down toward ground as a result of:
   1) the marked knee flexion
   2) the length of foot that protrudes beyond the line of the leg
   3) ankle in maximum equinis from assisting balance

RESPONSE:

Events	Anatomical Activity
FORWARD PROGRESSION:	
1. Entire extremity lifted to overcome postural and true equinus.	1. a. Active hip flexion (0° to 5°) by: iliacus, sartorius, tensor fascia femoris. b. Active knee flexion (50° to 70°) by: biceps femoris (short head), sartorius.
2. At toe-off, foot posterior and lateral to axis of body.	2. Extremity brought toward midline by adductor magnus.
LIMB LENGTH ADJUSTMENT:	
1. Limb shortened to aid toe clearance.	1. Pelvis rotates forward from its maximum posterior position.

THE MECHANICS OF WALKING

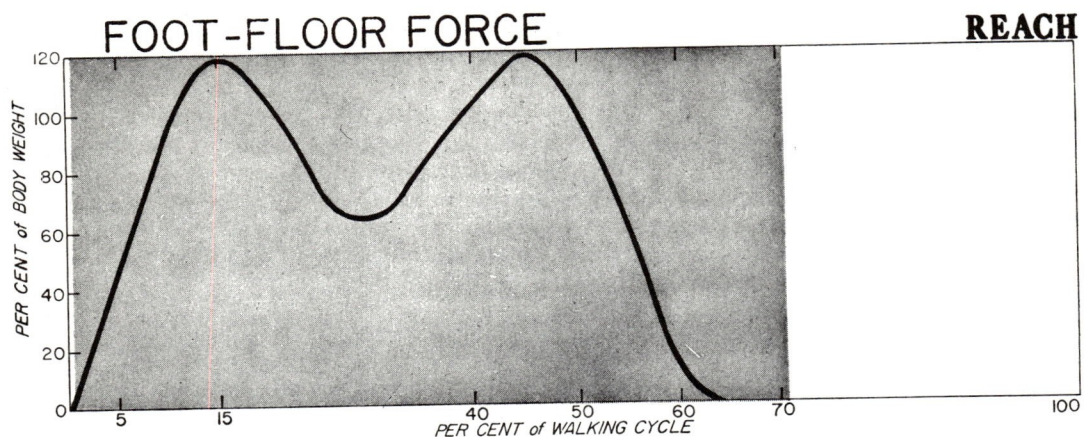

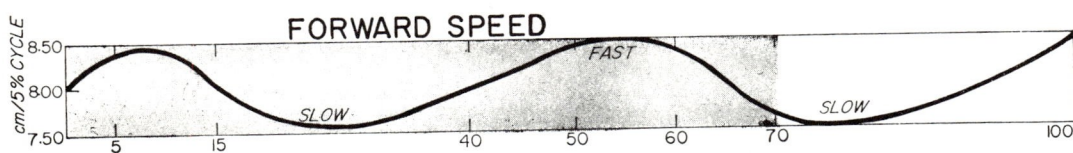

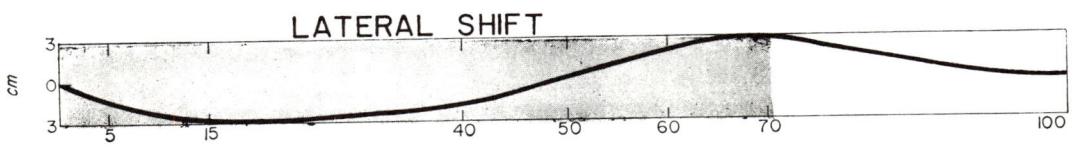

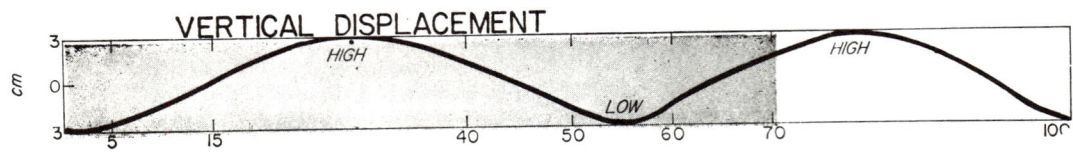

MUSCLE ACTION

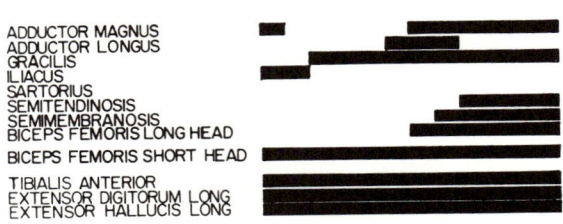

These graphs adapted from data published by Murray [7] and Cunningham.[12]

A CLINICAL INTERPRETATION

Plate 6. REACH

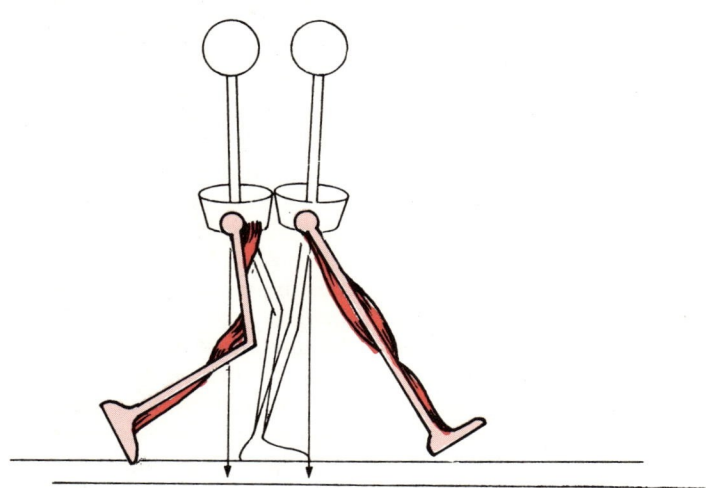

TASK: REACH (INTERVAL: LATE SWING)
   Period of Knee Extension During Swing: 75 to 100% of Walking Cycle

DEMAND:
   Advance foot for next step in forward progression.
   Be ready to receive the advancing body weight.

SITUATION:
   Body traveling forward as a result of previous push and stance activity of other limb.
   Extremity suspended in a flexed posture at every joint.
   Foot still behind axis of body.
   Toe clear.

RESPONSE:

Events	Anatomical Activity
FORWARD PROGRESSION:	
1. Limb advances rapidly to reach weight acceptance position before body weight is too far ahead for stability.	1. Knee extends rapidly from its 70 degrees flexed posture by relaxation of flexors and pendulum effect. Extensors (Vasti) become active at end of period to maintain full knee extension. Hip flexion increased slightly (to 30°) and maintained by adductors.
2. Toe kept clear of ground.	2. Active dorsiflexion.
LIMB LENGTH ADJUSTMENT:	
1. Limb lengthened.	1. Pelvis continues to rotate with advancing limb. Also drops into further adduction.

the hip is passively pushed into extension. Excessive strain of the anterior ligaments is avoided by the actions of the iliacus and adductor longus. As weight is just about to be transferred to the other foot, the body has returned to the midline and is preparing to shift to the other side. This lessens the demand on the hip abductors. At the same time the adductor magnus and adductor longus become active to control the shift medially.

Balance Assist

Almost immediately after the peak of the push-force, there is a rapid drop in the amount of weight being supported by that foot, yet the toe remains in contact with the ground. This is an interval of double limb support for the weight that is being rapidly transferred from one limb to the other (Plate 4). The continued contact with the floor by the toe of the limb that is discharging its weight, would seem to serve as a means of assisting in balance as the weight is being accepted by the other limb.

The knee flexes rapidly to a position of about 65 degrees. This appears to result largely from release of body weight on the taut gastrocnemius, as the gracilis is the only other flexor muscle active. Subsequent rectus femoris action at the end of this interval restrains the extent of flexion. It only reaches 70 degrees by the end of the next period.

At the same time as the knee is flexing rapidly, the hip is flexing at a more gradual rate as it recovers from the extended position. Again, the active musculature seems to be the adductors. They are probably providing the dual role of flexion as well as restraint of abduction as weight is being transferred across the midline to the other foot. During this interval of hip and knee flexion, toe contact is maintained by a proportional increase in ankle plantar flexion. The many plantar flexors are still active except for the gastrocnemius which has become silent. This extensive plantar flexion of about 20 degrees also serves to lengthen the limb relatively in spite of the marked knee flexion and the decrease in hip extension.

Clinically the significance rests with the ability of the person to have a graduated assist in balance as he transfers weight to the other side. When controlled plantar flexion is not available, the body weight has to be shifted at one time. The abrupt change in direction would be apparent as a limp, and it also would increase the work of the weight-accepting limb because of the increased impact of the exchange.

Pick-up

The final phases of forward progression relate to the forward swing of the limb (Plate 5). The extremity, relieved of its weight-bearing duties, is picked up and rapidly advanced from behind the body to in front of it.

Because the forefoot protrudes several inches beyond the anterior surface of the tibia, the toe is pointing down any time the hip is extended behind the body, unless there is extreme ankle dorsiflexion. This downward pointing is even greater when the knee is flexed. Thus, there is relative equinus of the foot even with the ankle in a neutral position.

Consequently, toe clearance is a combination of hip flexion, knee flexion and ankle dorsiflexion. It has always been difficult for investigators to determine the exact moment of toe-off because the decrease in ground force is a gradual lessening of contact during balance assist, and the amount of ground clearance is minimal. For maximum efficiency, no extra energy is expended and the toe just barely clears the ground by about a centimeter. At the same time, the hip and knee motions are smooth continuations of the postures started during the balance assist phase. The only real change is the abrupt shift from active plantar flexion while toe contact is being maintained to active dorsiflexion just after toe clearance has begun. The toe is prevented from dragging primarily by the continuance of the hip and knee flexion motions which lift the whole limb. By the end of the pick-up phase, the knee has flexed to a maximum 70 degrees. The hip and ankle are about midway in their flexion course. Because of the extensive knee flexion, the foot is still behind the line of the body.

Knee flexion is accomplished by the short head of the biceps femoris and the sartorius. The iliacus, sartorius, and tensor flex the hip. This is a significant interval clinically because the patient who has inadequate hip or knee flexion will drag his toe despite adequate ankle control. Thus the natural inclination to apply a short-leg brace to anyone who drags his toe must be restrained. During the period of pick-up, toe drag is due to the relative equinus of the foot and inadequate elevation of the entire extremity.

Inability to lift the extremity may be the result not only of paralytic difficulties, but also of restrictions of joint motion. The person who has considerable knee stiffness following prolonged immobilization for femoral shaft fractures, hip fusions, and so forth, must hike his pelvis to accommodate for this loss of motion. A fused hip would require even more knee flexion to clear the toe. Seldom do such patients have the excessive dorsiflexion that could substitute because the prolonged immobilization has included the ankle joint as well. Hence, an individual needs a minimum of 70 degrees to clear his toe on smooth ground, more on any rough terrain and over 100 degrees for negotiating stairs.

Reach

Having cleared the ground, the extremity is now stretched forward to prepare for the oncoming task of weight acceptance (Plate 6). This is accomplished by continuing hip flexion to a final position of 30 degrees. The so-called primary flexors of the hip which were active during pick-up are now silent even though hip flexion continues and is maintained. Undoubtedly much of this is momentum from the previous impetus but is also sustained by the gracilis, adductor longus and adductor magnus which are again active. Knee flexion is continued by the short head of the biceps femoris. There is a brief burst of rectus femoris activity at the end of the pick-up period just before the knee starts extending. The quadriceps are otherwise silent until the end of the reach when the vasti become active to maintain this extended posture in preparation for weight acceptance. At the same time the semimembranosus, semitendinosus and long head of the biceps become active, presumably to restrain the forward momentum of the limb at both the hip and knee. Hip flexion restraint assures a logical position for ground contact and knee restraint protects the ligaments from strain.

The foot attains a position of just less than neutral (5° equinus) and maintains it until heel strike. This is under the continued activity of the dorsiflexor muscles (tibialis anterior, extensor digitorum longus, extensor hallucis longus). The clinical problem of toe drop is now directly related to anterior ankle control.

The meagerness of muscular activity through this swing phase indicates the ease of swinging the extremity if there has been an adequate push-off. The greater magnitude of knee flexion range and knee flexor muscle activity, as compared to the hip, also indicates which area has the greatest need. This is borne out clinically for seldom need we be concerned about hip flexor activity unless the person lacks knee control as well. A further aid to clearing the foot is the fact that the weight is on the opposite leg and thus that side of the pelvis is relatively elevated even though it never comes above the horizontal.

As the extremity reaches forward, it is also being relatively lengthened by associated pelvic rotation and tilt (Fig. 4). In the course of the total swing phase from the moment of toe-off until the heel strikes once again, the extremity has recovered from relative lengthening to accommodate the posterior reach, attains its maximally shortened posture as it passes the vertical line and then again lengthens in order to reach forward. The pelvis both lifts and rotates forward as the limb advances to the midline. After this point the pelvis drops while it continues the forward rotation.

SUMMARY

The following points have the greatest clinical significance for normal walking.

1. As one starts to balance on one limb, there is a definite valgus thrust on the knee and foot as the individual shifts his weight on to the weight-bearing foot (Fig. 2).

2. By utilizing the pelvis as a means of increasing the relative length of the limb, the process of swinging one extremity from behind to forward carries the hip of the weight-bearing limb through adduction, internal rotation and extension while it is supporting full body weight (Fig. 4). Similar rotatory stresses are made on the knee and foot.

3. During the forward progression complex of actions, the single greatest factor preventing the knee from buckling on weight acceptance and trunk glide is control of the tibia through strong action of the plantar flexor muscles (Plate 1). The calf muscles must be strong or they must be replaced by contracture, fusion or bracing. Hip extensor control is the second significant factor. Direct quadriceps stabilization of the knee is the least important though, of course, very useful when present.

4. The body weight is advanced in front of the foot only if approximately 10 degrees of dorsiflexion is available (Plate 2). Otherwise, there will be a strong force to hyperextend the knee, and the hip must be able to support weight in flexion.

5. There is a postural equinus at the be-

ginning of the swing phase because the entire foot is tipped downward by the marked knee flexion that is present (Plate 5). Consequently, toe drag in this period is due to inadequate pick-up activity of the hip and knee flexors. Later, as the extremity reaches forward for the next step, continued toe drag would be the result of inadequate anterior ankle control.

CONCLUSION

Whenever the patient lacks the required joint range or muscle response (strength or timing), he will limp or have to exaggerate other actions to compensate for the deficiencies.

In treating patients the goal is safe, efficient ambulation. Encouragement to eliminate a limp or walking aid should be given only if the patient can afford the extra effort and tissue strain resulting from compensatory actions.

These goals for the patient can only be achieved if the physician and the therapist have a working knowledge of the mechanics of walking, and can apply these concepts to their evaluation and program planning for the individual patient and his specific problem.

REFERENCES

1. Eberhart, H. D., V. T. Inman, J. B. DeC. M. Saunders, A. S. Levens, B. Bresler and T. D. McCowan, Fundamental Studies of Human Locomotion and other Information Relating to the Design of Artificial Limbs. A Report to the National Research Council, Committee on Artificial Limbs. University of California, Berkeley, 1947.
2. Eberhart, H. D., V. T. Inman, and Boris Bresler, The Principal Elements in Human Locomotion, Chapter 15. In P. E. Klopsteg and P. D. Wilson: Human Limbs and Their Substitutes. McGraw-Hill Book Co., New York, 1954.
3. Saunders, J. B. DeC. M., V. T. Inman, and H. W. Eberhart, The Major Determinants in Normal and Pathological Gait. J. Bone Joint Surg., 35A:543–558, July 1953.
4. Elftman, H., A Cinematic Study of the Distribution of Pressure in the Human Foot. Anat. Record, 59:481–491, 1934.
5. Hubbard, A. W., and R. H. Stetson, An Experimental Analysis of Human Locomotion. Amer. J. Physiol., 124:300–314, 1938.
6. Schwartz, R. P., A. L. Heath, W. Mislek, and J. N. Wright, Kinetics of Human Gait. J. Bone Joint Surg., 16:343–350, 1934.
7. Murray, M. P., A. B. Drought, and R. C. Kory, Walking Patterns of Normal Men. J. Bone Joint Surg., 46A:335–360, 1964.
8. Murray, M. P., and B. H. Clarkson, The Vertical Pathways of the Foot During Level Walking: I. Range of Variability in Normal Men. J. Amer. Phys. Ther. Assoc., 46:585–589, 1966.
9. Sutherland, David H., An Electromyographic Study of the Plantar Flexors of the Ankle in Normal Walking on the Level. J. Bone Joint Surg., 48A:66–71, January 1966.
10. Close, J. R. and F. N. Todd, The Phasic Activity of the Muscles of the Lower Extremity and the Effect of Tendon Transfer. J. Bone Joint Surg., 41A:189–208, 1959.
11. The Pattern of Muscular Activity in the Lower Extremity During Walking. A Presentation of Summarized Data. Prosthetic Devices Research, Institute of Engineering Research, University of California, Berkeley. Series II, Issue 25, September 1953.
12. Cunningham, D. M., Components of Floor Reactions During Walking. Prosthetic Devices Research Project, Institute of Engineering Research, University of California, Berkeley. Series II, Issue 14, November 1950 (Reissued, October 1958)

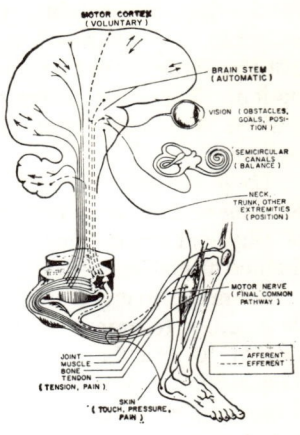

RELATIONSHIP BETWEEN LESION SPECIFICITY AND BRACING

JACQUELIN PERRY, M.D.

Normal walking has specific requirements of co-ordination, muscular strength, and joint mobility. Whenever physical impairment renders these functions less than adequate, the patient's ability to walk is threatened. Under these circumstances the minimal goals are to maintain or acquire adequate stability to remain erect, and sufficient mobility to take steps in sequence. Smoothness of gait and efficiency of effort are sacrificed.

The necessary stability can be gained through bracing, hence, with sufficient apparatus every person can stand. But for effective walking, the brace must also permit the patient to utilize his remaining function so as to have the mobility to take the necessary steps. Disruption in mobility-stability balance varies with the type of physical impairment of the patient, and consequently brace design must also vary with the nature of the lesion.

A brace provides stability, or the correction of deformity, by rigidly or selectively restricting motion, by spring assistance to weakened muscles, and by the stimulation of reflex responses through skin pressure which gives proprioceptive clues. The key to gaining the advantages of braces without unduly restricting the patient's mobility, rests with selecting the appropriate method of providing the required stability. This in turn depends on whether the physical lesion is a disturbance of muscle, joint, nerve, spinal cord or brain.

In concentrating on the functional loss evidenced at the periphery, the difference in the mechanism of disability is often forgotten. For example, the equinus found in poliomyelitis is not the same as the equinus seen in the stroke patient. The spring assist which helps the polio patient will only aggravate hemiplegic spasticity.

To overcome this failing, this discussion of bracing techniques will focus on the actual sites of physical impairment and the way they influence function.

To make even a single motion, there must be a motor to create the activity and a leverage system to translate this activity into motion. The human motor is muscle, and the minimal leverage system consists of two bones with a functioning joint between them. If the muscle were not connected to levers such as these, its contraction would be merely an isolated electro-chemical phenomenon and a bulge under the skin.

The physiological dependence of the muscle fiber on its motor neuron makes it more appropriate to consider the entire motor unit as the source of motion rather than focusing just on muscle (Fig. 1). The motor unit consists of the anterior horn cell lying within the spinal

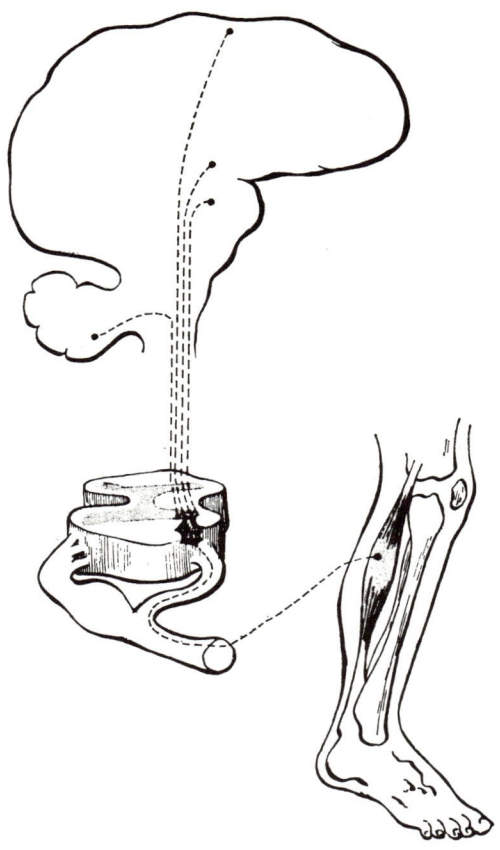

FIG. 2. Motor control signals arising from centers within the cerebral cortex, brain stem, or cerebellum, instruct the appropriate motor units when to become active. The instructions for action may be initiated as a selected voluntary motion, as a primitive synergy, or as part of a highly complex, learned co-ordination pattern.

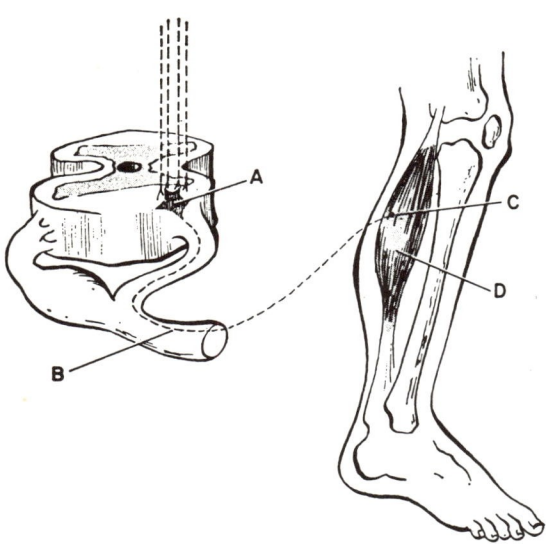

FIG. 1. The motor unit is the final common pathway that translates all instructions into motion. Its components are: (A) anterior horn cell, (B) alpha motor neuron (peripheral nerve), (C) myoneural junction, and (D) muscle. Dysfunction of any one of these components blocks all action of the unit. Each alpha motor neuron branches to supply from 10 to 1,000 muscle fibers depending upon the character of the individual muscle.

cord, the alpha neurons in the peripheral nerve, the myoneural junction and the muscle fibers. Disruption of any one of these components will prevent the production of motion, for the muscle fiber is inert without its appropriate motor nerve signals.

Incorporation of this motion into a purposeful task requires central motor control to provide the specific instructions of when to move, how much to move, and how long to continue moving—with such instructions going to several muscles to accomplish the numerous actions and restraints needed to complete the task (Fig. 2). The initial attempt at this co-ordinated motion may be considered as a calculated guess of what is necessary. If the result is satisfactory, the same pattern will be followed again. If not, it will be modified to seek

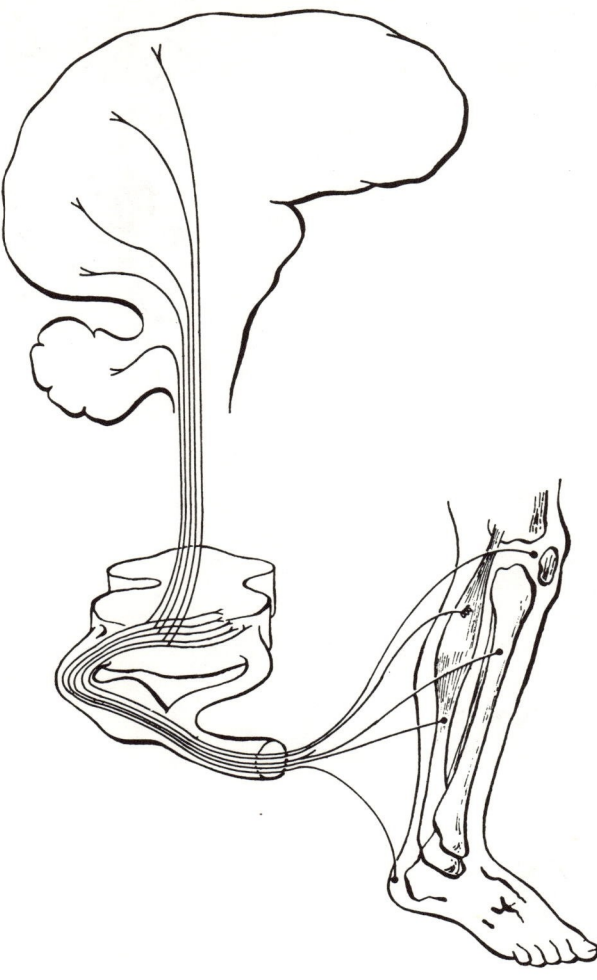

FIG. 3. The sensory pathways, both peripheral and central, are the key to motion as an individual does not know what his next move should be unless he is aware of his current position and the effects of the last motor instructions.

a better result. The indications of how to modify and the need to modify, arise from the guiding sensory system (Fig. 3). This consists of the ability to receive sensations and the ability to interpret these sensations into meaningful motor directions.

Walking is obviously a complex purposeful task and requires normal function of each component to attain the usual smooth efficient pattern of action. The essential components for motion are listed in Table 1.

As a result of disease or injury, these systems can be damaged singly or in various combinations. Bracing techniques to compensate for the resulting abnormal performance must vary appropriately.

TABLE 1

ESSENTIALS FOR PURPOSEFUL FUNCTION

Motor Units
Leverage Systems
Sensory Reception
Sensory Interpretation
Central Motor Control

It is now evident that effective treatment of the patient, and effective bracing, depend upon awareness of the level of disability, on developing ways to utilize that which remains and to substitute for that which is lost.

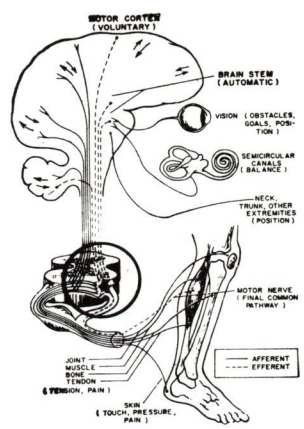

PARALYTIC DYSFUNCTION

I. Pathomechanics

JACQUELIN PERRY, M.D.

MOTOR UNIT DISORDERS

OF THE MANY systems involved in purposeful activities, the most easily managed with bracing is disruption of the motor system because it results in a flaccid paralysis. The motor unit has four distinctive areas where it can be damaged by disease. The anterior horn cell within the spinal cord is the victim of the poliomyelitis virus. Infectious neuronitis attacks the axons. The myoneural junction is the selective site of myasthenia gravis, while muscular dystrophy isolates its destruction to the muscle fibers. The principles of bracing would be the same for these four types of disability, though the general course of illness usually restricts the use of braces to patients with polio and muscular dystrophy. For simplicity, the discussion of techniques regarding this variety of bracing has been focused on two disabilities, poliomyelitis and low spinal cord injuries. The principles apply equally well, however, to any other form of motor unit disruption.

The primary characteristic of poliomyelitis is the purity of the lesion. Sensory reception, sensory interpretation and motor control are normal in patients with residual disability.

Only the motor unit system has been disturbed. This means that the patient disabled by poliomyelitis has a precise sense of position, appropriate judgment of action, and precise control of all the musculature that is still innervated. The efficient utilization of his remaining musculature has established standards of performance which cannot be matched by patients with disturbances of any of the other systems.

Intact position sense also allows the polio patient to substitute postural stability for lost muscle action. In other words, by changing his body alignment he can rest against taut ligaments for joint support. This provides him with a substituting mechanism unavailable to persons with even minor disturbances of motor control or sensory function.

Disturbance of walking due to a spinal cord injury has been included in the paralytic group. This has been done because the patient with a cord injury who becomes an effective walker is the patient with a flaccid paralysis; a person with a limited motor lesion similar to that seen in poliomyelitis.

The lumbar and sacral nerves that innervate the muscles of the lower extremities lie compressed in the distal end of the spinal cord. This area is the span of the first lumbar vertebra and its disk, a common site for fracture. The tearing or crushing of the cord that accompanies the vertebral injury causes direct damage to the anterior horn cells which supply the motor nerves to the muscles of the lower limb. A flaccid paralysis results which is similar to that observed in poliomyelitis.

However, similar motor losses from spinal cord injury and from polio do not leave the patients with the same ability to walk. The polio virus invades only the anterior horn cells, whereas the traumatic lesion disrupts the entire cross section of the cord. As a result, the sensory axons which bring in the signals from the periphery have also been damaged. This loss of sensory reception from the lower extremities denies the spinal cord injury patient the precise awareness of position that permits fine changes in body alignment to attain postural stability. His substitutions of ligamentous tension for muscular support are quite gross, as his sensory clues come from more distant sources: trunk, eyes, and balance center in the central nervous system.

CORD CONTROL DISORDERS

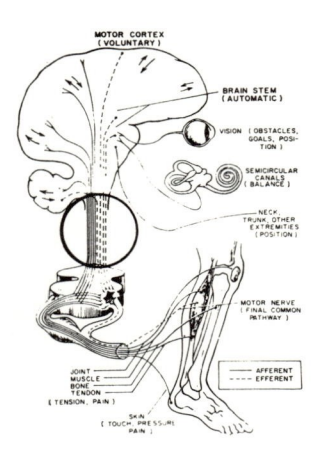

When the spinal cord injury occurs above the lumbar segments, the neurological picture and the potential to walk change abruptly. Rather than the relatively simple picture of a flaccid paralysis with an associated sensory loss, there is now loss of motor control and spasticity is present—far more difficult problems to manage.

The thoracic level lesion interrupts the tracts that carry the co-ordinated motor instructions down from the brain, and similarly, prevents the sensory signals of the lower extremity from reaching the brain's interpretive centers.

At the same time, the motor unit and sensory receptive pathways below the level of the injury are undisturbed, that is, they are normal. The preservation of these reflex arcs with concommitant loss of control creates the mechanism of spasticity.

The area of local damage occurring within the thoracic spine also involves the anterior horn cells and sensory receptor terminals at the level of the lesion. In the lower thoracic segments this means there will be paralysis of the abdominals, and hence less trunk stability. Higher thoracic lesions will limit the flaccid area to the appropriate intercostal muscles; but the abdominal muscles, having lost their control and released the mechanism of spasticity, are again unable to give adequate trunk stability. Thus, the person with a thoracic lesion is a poor candidate for walking.

II. Bracing the Unstable Knee in Flaccid Paralysis

MARILYN J. LISTER, B.S.

The patient with flaccid paralysis who needs a long-leg brace for knee stability can be fitted with one of two kinds of braces: a free-knee brace with an eccentric knee joint, or a conventional long-leg brace. Both braces can stabilize the knee, and it is the role of the physical therapist to analyze which brace can best solve the individual patient's problem.

It is necessary to know the specific purpose for the brace and what the patient is able to do to meet the requirements of the brace in order to make the appropriate choice.

THE FREE-KNEE BRACE

The free-knee brace has no intrinsic locking mechanism (Fig. 1). It is designed to restrict knee motion just during stance, which is the only time a force is needed to prevent the knee from buckling. During the swing phase of gait it offers no resistance to flexion.

The eccentric knee joint of the brace produces knee stability by relying on the body weight's being in front of the joint (Fig. 2). Any position which causes the body weight to fall behind the eccentric joint will unlock the knee and create instability.

The free-knee brace also relies on the ankle joint's being limited to 90 degrees of dorsiflexion with about 10 degrees of plantar flexion allowed to permit the foot to go flat at heel strike.

The UCLA Brace

The concept of this free-knee brace is similar to that of the one designed at UCLA.[1] The uniqueness of the "UCLA" brace is the design of the ankle and the use of a quadrilateral plastic thigh cuff. The purpose of their ankle unit is to retain the advantages of the tibial control gained by a locked ankle, yet eliminate the forward thrust that occurs at heel–strike because of the restriction of ankle plantar flexion.

BRACING THE FLACCID KNEE

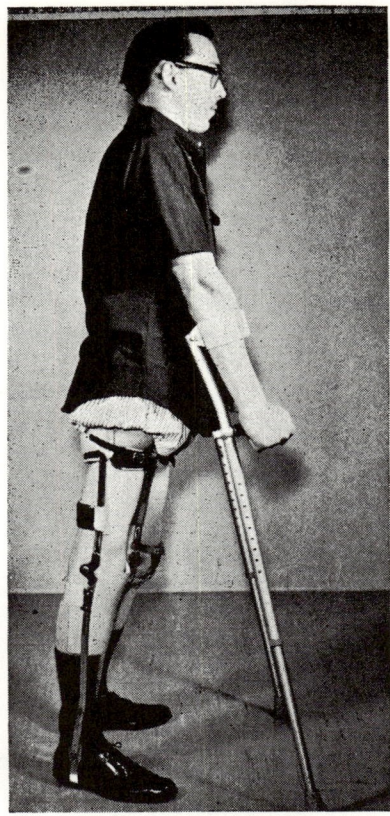

FIG. 1. The free-knee brace with eccentric knee joint and no intrinsic locking mechanism.

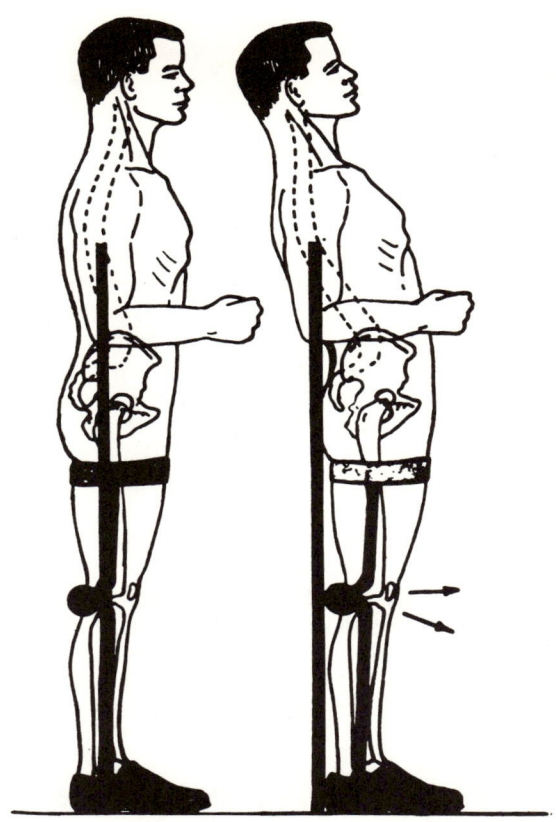

FIG. 2. The eccentric joint of the free-knee brace relies on the body weight being in front of the joint (left) in order to be locked. Any position which causes the body weight to fall behind the eccentric knee joint (right) will unlock the knee.

The unit consists of two hydraulic pistons which allow the ankle to plantar flex, but resist dorsiflexion as the tibia advances with forward momentum. Dorsiflexion beyond 90 degrees is prevented.

The concept is excellent, but the unit as currently designed has several disadvantages. Because the pistons are located at the ankle, they are conspicuous and make it difficult for boys to pull their trousers over their braces. Also, they are subject to the dirt and grime of the streets and thus difficult to keep operational.

The biggest disadvantage, however, is the fact that the added weight at the end of the extremity slows the rate at which the leg swings forward to a stable "reach" position. Consequently, the patient must walk at a slower pace as he waits for the foot to get ahead of the body.

This follows the well-established principle of pendulum action which notes that the greater the weight at its end, the slower will be its arc of motion. The leg swinging from the knee acts like a pendulum as there is no active control for knee extension.

The UCLA quadrilateral thigh cuff was designed to reproduce the stability offered by the prosthetic quadrilateral socket. While it does provide excellent stability, it is difficult for patients to apply and the weight (approximately 4 pounds) is an excessive load on the severely paralyzed hip.

As a means of utilizing the principle, but offsetting the disadvantages, we have substituted a contoured metal cuff weighing about 4 ounces. Clinical experience has demonstrated that the patient gets adequate stability from this lighter thigh cuff.

Only an occasional patient has found the graduated dorsiflexion restraint unit of sufficient value to accept its limitations. Others find the locked ankle joint satisfactory. It is hoped, however, that a new design will make this concept practical.

Candidates for the Free-Knee Brace

A patient is a candidate for a free-knee brace if his paralysis is unilateral, if his trunk can balance over the hip while his body weight falls in front of the eccentric knee joint of the brace, and if his foot is stable. This type of patient can usually walk without a brace if he uses his hand against his thigh to push the knee back into extension for knee stability, or if he minimizes weight bearing by hopping quickly over the involved extremity. Walking in this manner consumes large amounts of energy, is cosmetically undesirable, is often unsafe, and limits the use of the hands for other functions. Provided with a free-knee brace to give knee stability, this patient can walk independently and safely without crutches or canes. In essence, this means the person is normal except for severe paralysis of one lower extremity and this extremity is free from deformity.

The three essentials necessary for a patient to use a free-knee brace are (Fig. 3): (1) near vertical hip-trunk alignment, (2) absence of knee flexion contracture, and (3) a foot that rests flat on the floor.

Near Vertical Hip-Trunk Alignment. The ability of the patient to attain near vertical hip-trunk alignment is dependent upon his trunk strength, hip strength, and the range of motion of the hip joint. If there is inadequate strength of the hip extensor muscles, the patient must have sufficient trunk control to compensate for the lack of hip stability by leaning backward (Fig. 4). The degree of trunk hyperextension permissible to gain hip stability is minimal to keep the body weight in front of the eccentric knee joint.

Effective hip-trunk alignment is possible for the patient with Zero strength of the hip extensor muscles if there is full passive range of motion in hip extension.

If, however, there is a slight (10–15°) hip flexion deformity (Fig. 5), the hip extensor

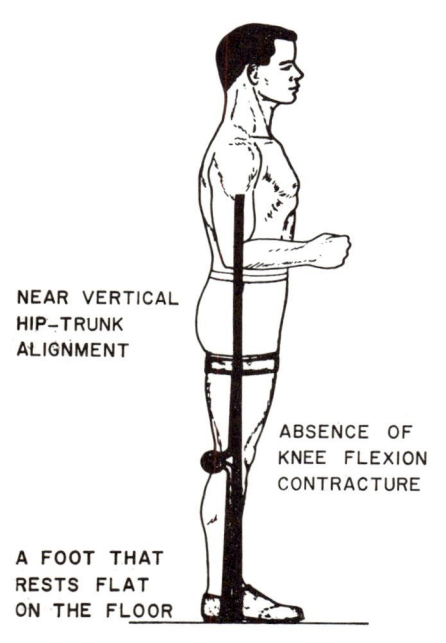

FIG. 3. Requirements for a patient to use a free-knee brace.

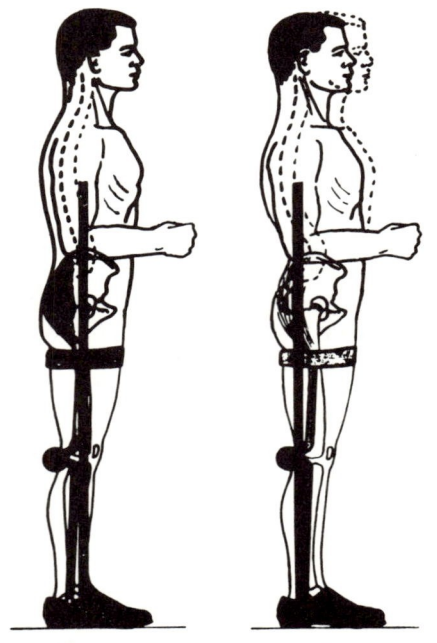

FIG. 4. A patient with adequate strength of the hip extensor muscles (left) can attain near vertical hip–trunk alignment. A patient with inadequate hip extensor strength (right) must have sufficient trunk control to compensate for the lack of hip stability by leaning backward a minimal amount.

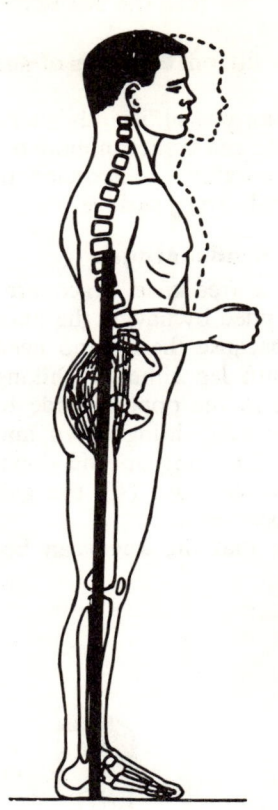

BRACING THE FLACCID KNEE

muscle strength must be at least Poor in order to maintain such balance. An even greater flexion deformity demands a great deal more extensor strength.

The common physical findings which prevent hip-trunk alignment are: (1) hip flexion deformity without adequate hip extensor strength to lock the hip (Fig. 6A); (2) unopposed active muscular force which pulls the hip into flexion (Fig. 6A); (3) a hip that requires the trunk to lean too far back in order to be stable, thereby placing the body weight behind the eccentric knee joint (Fig. 6B).

Absence of Knee Fexion Contracture. Full passive range of motion in knee extension is needed so the knee can be placed in a stable position and the extremity can be placed in proper alignment. Five degrees of hyperextension range in the knee is even more desirable (Fig. 7). This will permit the anatomical knee joint to increase its normal eccentric function and allow greater stability during weight bearing. A knee flexion deformity decreases stability at the knee as well as indirectly

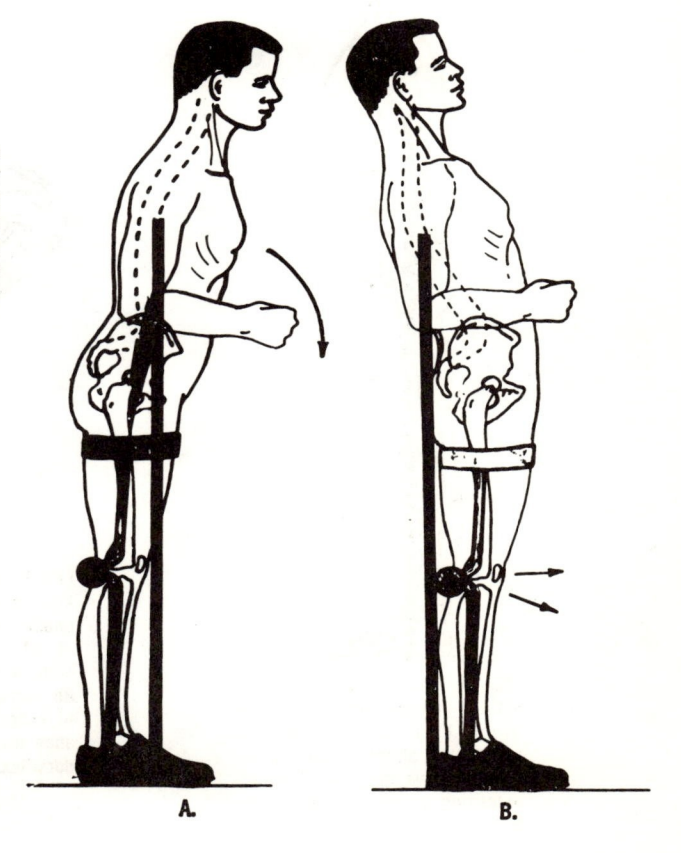

FIG. 5. The patient with a slight (10-15°) hip flexion deformity needs at least Poor hip extensor muscle strength to maintain balance. Note resulting lordosis when patient is balanced.

FIG. 6. (A) Hip–trunk alignment is prevented by a hip flexion deformity without adequate hip extensor strength, or by unopposed active muscular force which pulls the hip into flexion. (B) Alignment is also prevented by a hip that requires the trunk to lean too far back in order to be stable, thereby placing the body weight behind the eccentric knee joint.

causing hip flexion because of the obliquity of the femur (Fig. 8). The patient will not be able to balance with the ankle joint of the brace locked at 90 degrees because the knee flexion deformity causes the body weight to fall too far behind the eccentric knee joint. Also, an excessive amount of hip flexion is created in an attempt to keep the body weight in front of the knee joint.

A Foot that Rests Flat on the Floor. The patient cannot rest his foot flat on the floor in a stable position for weight bearing if the foot is deformed.

An equinus contracture of more than 5–10 degrees will also prevent the patient from using a free-knee brace because it indirectly causes hip and knee flexion by relatively lengthening the limb (Fig. 9). The only way to avoid this is with a full-sole lift on the shoe of the good leg.

If the involved extremity is sufficiently short, the degree of contracture can be accommodated by a shoe lift that is carefully constructed to provide a stable weight-bearing surface.

Advantages and Disadvantages

The advantages of a free-knee brace are: (1) less energy is expended by having the knee bend during walking because there is no need to compensate for a stiff leg either by hiking the hip, or by leaning to the opposite side to advance the extremity; (2) sitting down and standing up is easier; (3) going up and down stairs is done with greater ease; (4) the gait is more normal in appearance.

The disadvantage is that the knee can be-

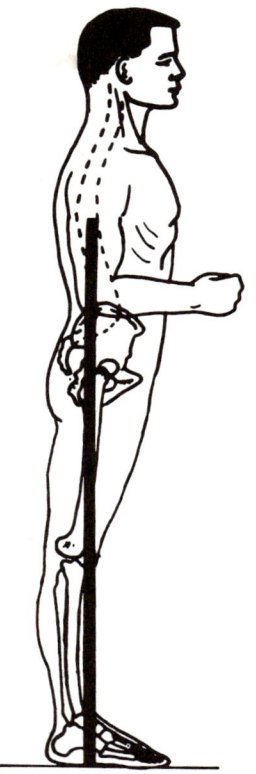

FIG. 7. Full passive range of motion in knee extension is required to allow knee stability and proper alignment of the extremity. Five degrees of hyperextension is even more desirable.

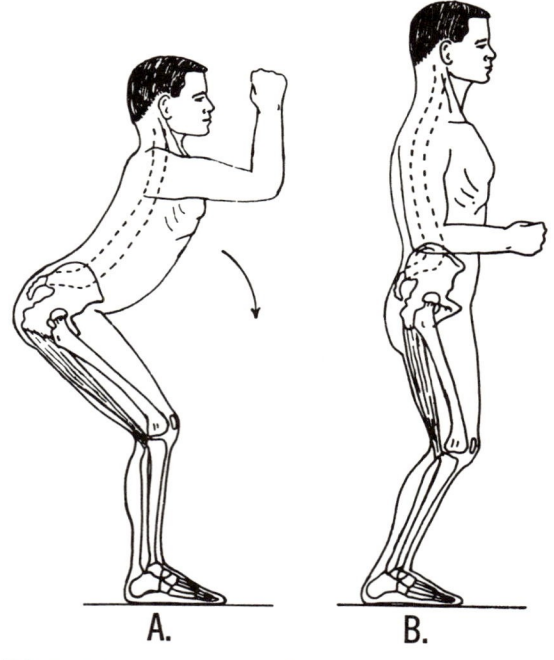

FIG. 8. A knee flexion deformity decreases stability at the knee and indirectly causes hip flexion. (A) The patient is unable to balance with the ankle joint of the brace locked at 90 degrees because knee flexion deformity causes the body weight to fall too far behind the eccentric knee joint. An excessive amount of hip flexion is created in an attempt to keep the body weight in front of the knee joint. (B) Balance would be possible if the patient were permitted some dorsiflexion.

BRACING THE FLACCID KNEE

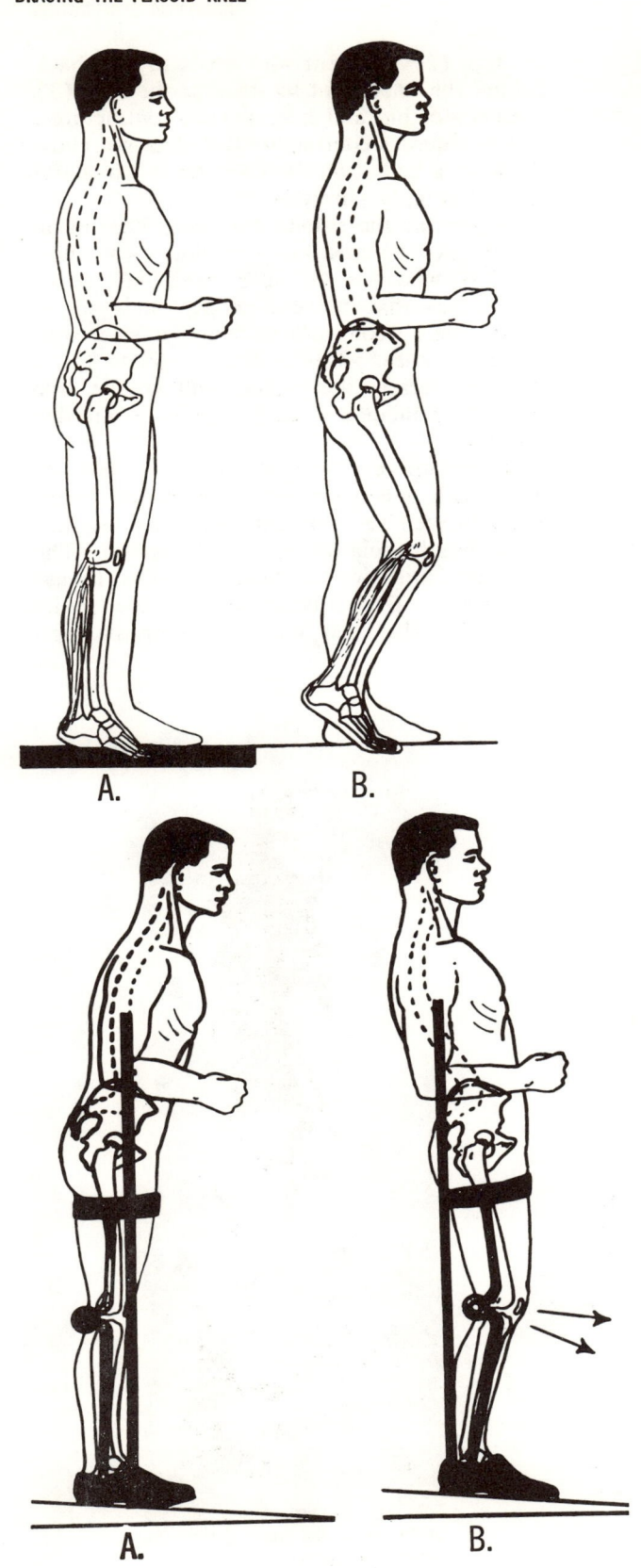

FIG. 9. (A) An equinus contracture will lengthen the limb relatively. (B) Weight bearing on a foot with an equinus contracture of more than 5–10 degrees will indirectly cause hip and knee flexion, thereby preventing the patient from using a free-knee brace.

FIG. 10. A disadvantage of the free-knee brace is knee instability when walking down an incline, if the patient has difficulty with trunk balance. (A) The patient has adequate strength to balance trunk while going down an incline. (B) The patient without adequate strength in the hip and trunk must lean back over the hip for stability. His body weight is then placed behind the eccentric knee joint which causes the knee to buckle.

the hip; (2) a patient who needs to lean back behind the knee joint to stabilize the hip; (3) presence of hip and knee flexion contractures; (4) an equinus contracture that does not allow the foot to be flat on the floor; or (5) bilateral lower-extremity paralysis.

In general, the patient who must depend on exaggerated compensatory motion to stabilize the hip, who has unstable trunk balance or deformities that prevent proper body alignment, needs a conventional long-leg brace with a locked knee. Unlike the candidate for a free-knee brace, this patient will not be able to walk without a brace, even in a guarded fashion.

There are very few patients who cannot be fitted with a conventional locked-knee brace, though excessive knee and foot deformity may make weight bearing intolerably painful. The problems arise in the patient's ability to use the brace. Brace usage requires the ability to balance the head and trunk over the hips,

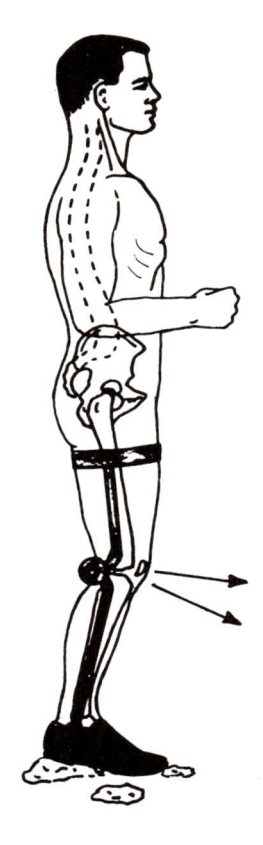

FIG. 11. Walking over an uneven surface may not be possible for the patient who has difficulties with trunk balance but who wears a free-knee brace. If the heel lands on a rock, or if the forefoot falls into a hole or depression, the knee will be forced into flexion and the body weight will shift behind the eccentric knee joint, causing the knee to buckle.

come unstable when walking down an incline (Fig. 10) or over an uneven surface (Fig. 11) if the patient has difficulty with trunk balance. Also, the speed of walking is restricted as the patient must wait for pendulum action to advance the leg. This is similar to the problem of the amputee, but the braced limb is heavier.

THE LOCKED-KNEE BRACE

The conventional long-leg brace (Fig. 12) which locks the knee during the entire gait cycle is indicated for patients who cannot use a free-knee brace as described. Several indications for the locked-knee brace are: (1) a trunk too weak or unstable to balance over

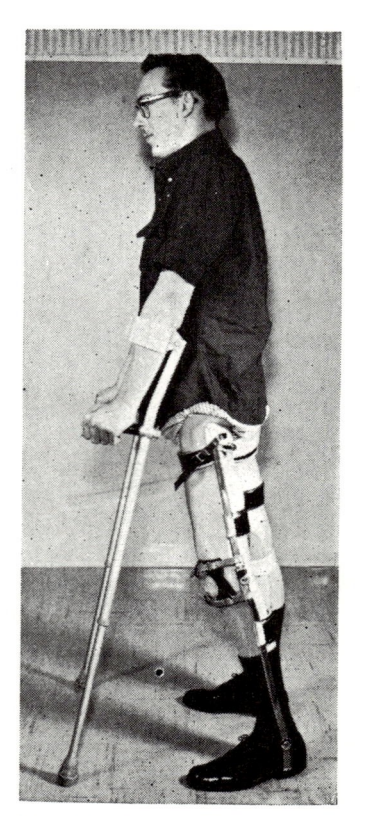

FIG. 12. A conventional long-leg brace locks the knee during the entire gait cycle.

balance on one foot, move forward, and the patient must be able to endure the extra energy expenditure required.

To accomplish the necessary balance in the long-leg, locked-knee brace, the patient must be able to lean backward over the hip for stability or use crutches for assistance.

Deformity is the biggest problem that prevents the patient from walking in a locked-knee brace. Hip or knee flexion deformities, or an equinus contracture, will prevent walking unless the patient's arms and trunk have sufficient muscular strength to maintain the essential trunk and hip stability.

Respiratory inadequacy can also interfere with ambulation. The respiratory problem may be too severe for the work that is required. Glossopharyngeal breathing is an excellent method of supplementing diminished breathing and improving the endurance of the patient.[2]

The advantages of the conventional locked-knee brace are knee stability when walking on any surface, and accommodation of the brace to a flexion contracture of moderate degree.

The disadvantages are the requirement that the patient compensate for a "stiff leg" to advance the limb during walking, and the additional energy expenditure.

The conventional long-leg brace can also be used to support weak or damaged ligamentous structures of the knee even if the patient does not have loss of muscular strength. In such instances, the knee joint of the brace can be left unlocked. An example of the need for ligamentous protection is a genu recurvatum problem in the growing child.

PHYSICAL THERAPY PROGRAM

The physical therapy program for the patient who needs a long-leg brace can be planned in two stages: preparation and functional training. The first stage is planned to prevent deformity, to stretch undesirable contractures, if present, and to strengthen the essential muscles. The second stage is gait training and a maintenance program.

Prevention of Deformity

The most important objective of physical therapy is to prevent deformity. For optimum functional use of either variety of long-leg brace, the patient must have full range of hip and knee extension and not more than 5 degrees of equinus contracture. The patient

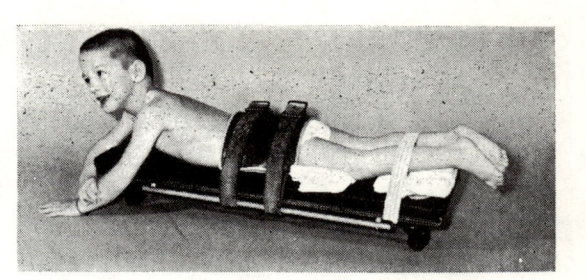

FIG. 13. A "prone board" allows the patient to be mobile while maintaining the prone position.

can tolerate 10 to 15 degrees of hip flexion if he has adequate hip extensor strength, but this consumes energy and results in decreased walking ability.

A positioning program must be planned to prevent the formation of contractures since passive range of motion done a few times daily is not adequate.

The patient's tendency to develop hip flexion contractures determines the amount of time he should be permitted to be in the flexed position, either sitting or lying curled up. Such control over his position is not always easy to accomplish.

When walking is difficult for the patient, he will probably walk only short distances and sit for the remainder of his waking hours. Lying supine in bed in full extension does not prevent flexion deformities because most beds are soft enough to permit at least 15 degrees of hip flexion. The patient must be placed in the prone position.

Some patients are able to prevent hip flexion contractures just by sleeping prone at night. Others need to lie prone for short periods during the day as well. Patients tolerate the prone position during their waking hours with more ease if they can be mobile on such devices as the prone guerney or the prone board (Fig. 13).

Correction of Deformity

If hip and knee flexion contractures already exist, a stretching program must be added to correct these deformities. Static stretch (Fig. 14) to the hips and knees should be carried out two times a day for thirty minutes on each extremity.

This must be followed by a progressive prone positioning program. The prone position is continually adjusted to keep up with

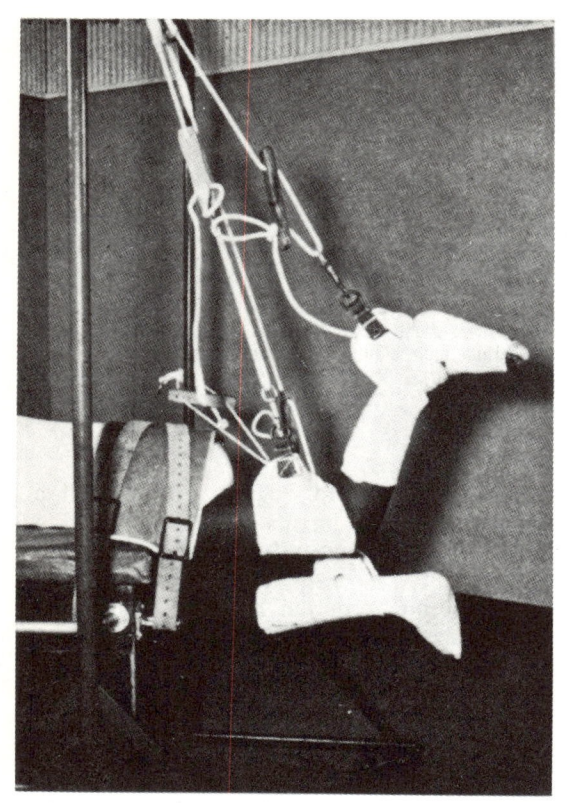

FIG. 14. The hip is placed on a static stretch in order to reduce a hip flexion contracture.

the patient's gain in range of motion. The maximum program is a twenty-four hour period in the prone position with fifteen-minute rest periods every two to three hours. Again, the patient is allowed to remain mobile during the day on the prone guerney and prone board. The patient is not permitted to resume sitting functions until the deformities are corrected.

The tendo calcaneus is stretched, if indicated, but 5 degrees of equinus should be retained. This tightness gives additional control by preventing the tibia from moving forward at the ankle during weight bearing thereby adding extension stability to the knee.

Any existing tightness in the hip abductor muscles is stretched except for a residual 10-degree contracture. The patient usually does not have abduction strength and will need slight tightness of the abductors for lateral stability.

If there is weakness in the back musculature, any residual tightness is maintained as an aid to stability in the upright position. If stretched out, the patient may not be a candidate for walking unless trunk stability can be achieved by surgical procedures or adequate external support.

The rib cage may also require stretching to improve breathing function. Chest cage mobility may be maintained by using intermittent positive pressure.

Improving Muscular Strength

The strengthening program depends on the available musculature. Progressive resistive exercise is started on the key groups: shoulder depressors, elbow extensors, trunk, hip extensors, hip abductors, quadriceps, and gastrocnemius muscles. This program is initiated even if the muscles have been graded as Poor.

The respiratory muscles may also need progressive resistive exercise. One example of this is placing weights on the epigastric area in order to strengthen the diaphragm.

Teaching Function

Functional training is started before the prescribed brace is received by using padded posterior wooden splints. Balance training is most essential. The patient must learn how to shift his trunk over the involved hip to gain stability, and how to use body momentum to advance his leg.

Patients with gluteus medius weakness who wear either kind of brace can improve their gait by using a cane in the opposite hand.[3] The lateral trunk motion almost disappears when the center of gravity does not have to shift to compensate for inadequate hip abduction.

Maintaining Function

Part of the training on how to use a long-leg brace includes teaching the patient how to stay in condition to wear the appliance. Emphasis is placed on preventing hip and knee flexion contractures and a home program is planned with the patient. The instructions include a specific positioning program as well as a maintenance exercise program. The gastroc-soleus muscles can usually be kept free from contracture by minimal daily walking, plus the protection afforded by wearing the brace all day. Unless the patient is an exceptionally active walker, he will probably spend most of the day sitting. It is the responsibility of the physical therapist to teach and "sell" the patient that only prevention of deformity will keep him ambulatory and functional.

SUMMARY

Many patients with unilateral flaccid paralysis need a long-leg brace for knee stability. The two kinds of braces commonly used are a free-knee brace and a conventional long-leg brace with a locked knee.

A patient is a candidate for a free-knee brace if he can balance the trunk directly over the hip or obtain hip stability with such a minimal amount of hyperextension that his body weight still lies in front of the eccentric knee joint.

A patient who has some ability to balance is a candidate for a conventional long-leg brace even though he cannot meet the critical requirement of trunk balance necessary for using the free-knee brace.

The greatest limiting factor in the functional use of either brace is a hip or knee flexion deformity.

The physical therapy program is planned to:
- Prevent deformity.
- Stretch undesirable contractures.
- Strengthen essential muscle groups.
- Provide functional training in the use of the brace.
- Establish a home program that will keep the patient walking.

Acknowledgement is given to Jane Lightfoot, B.S., Department of Physical Therapy, Rancho Los Amigos Hospital, who did the illustrations for this paper.

REFERENCES

1. Strohm, Bernard R., John Bray, and Sam C. Colachis, Jr., Check-out, Evaluation and Clinical Experience of the U.C.L.A. Functional Long Leg Brace. J. Amer. Phys. Ther. Ass., 46:829–834, August 1966.
2. Dail, C. W., J. E. Affeldt, and C. R. Collier, Clinical Aspects of Glossopharyngeal Breathing; Report of use by One Hundred Postpoliomyelitic Patients. J.A.M.A., 158:445–449, June 11, 1955.
3. Blount, Walter P., Don't Throw Away the Cane. J. Bone Joint Surg., 38A:695–708, June, 1956.

III. Brace Design for Flaccid Paralysis

DAVID HEIZER, C.O.

The two types of long-leg braces available to the orthotist are the locked-knee brace and the free-knee brace.

THE LOCKED-KNEE BRACE

The conventional means of supporting the unstable knee is use of a brace locked in extension throughout the walking cycle, but which can be released for sitting (Fig. 1, right). The essentials are two vertical bars and three points of fixation: a high posterior thigh cuff, an anterior knee control, and the shoe. In addition, the brace has an anterior thigh strap to hold it against the upper portion of the thigh and three bands (one above and two below the knee) to add stability to the brace. More extensive support, such as laced cuffs or a pretibial shell, is indicated only when there is structural insufficiency of either the bones or the joints.

In the past, there have been sporadic attempts to lessen the weight of the brace by utilizing a single lateral bar to eliminate the problem of the medial bars catching on each other. However, the resulting torque and instability make the single bar design unsafe for walking. Careful selection of the materials for construction is a more appropriate way of minimizing the weight of the brace and still attaining sufficient strength for safety and long-life expectancy.

The bars of the brace are made of aluminum and for the average adult, a $5/8$- x $3/16$-inch bar is adequate.

The choice of stirrup and its method of attachment to the shoe varies with the type of ankle joint needed by the patient. The free ankle joint, with or without a dorsiflexion assist, has no special requirement. If ankle motion is to be limited, stainless steel rivets should be used to attach the stirrup to the brace, as the more usual copper rivet will stretch and break making the brace useless.

Knee Joint Locks

Two basic styles of knee joint locks are available: drop locks and bail locks. Drop locks offer maximum security, but they must be placed and released manually. Small ball bearing catches make the task somewhat easier as they hold the lock up out of the way after they have been released.

The bail lock catches automatically when the knee joint is fully extended and is released by pulling up on the bail. This can be done by hitting the bail on the back of the chair, an action which becomes an almost automatic part of the patient's sitting motion. To avoid having the bail elevate inadvertently, an elastic strap is often used between the bail and the calf cuff. The stability of the bail decreases with time as the joint wears.

THE ECCENTRIC FREE-KNEE BRACE

The eccentric free-knee brace offers the patient the opportunity of flexing the knee during the swing phase of gait while providing necessary stability during stance (Fig. 1, left). The three points of fixation needed to lock the knee during stance are: pressure on the anterior thigh strap, an offset knee joint, and a 90-degree dorsiflexion stop.

Ankle Joints

Three types of ankle joints have been utilized in the free-knee brace. The locked ankle offers maximum stability of the tibia. However, at the moment of heel strike, the lack of plantar flexion throws the tibia forward, exaggerating the tendency to knee flexion. This tendency is partially offset by limitation of dorsiflexion and by momentum which is carrying the thigh forward. Nevertheless, stability is less than ideal with the locked ankle joint.

A more stable design which avoids the problem of forward ankle thrust is a carefully balanced limited-range ankle joint. There should be sufficient plantar flexion (about 10 degrees) for the foot to go flat at heel strike and dorsiflexion should be restricted to 90 degrees. Undesired toe drag is avoided by a weak dorsiflexion spring-assist—one which just lifts the foot but is not strong enough to interfere with the foot's going into plantar flexion at heel strike.

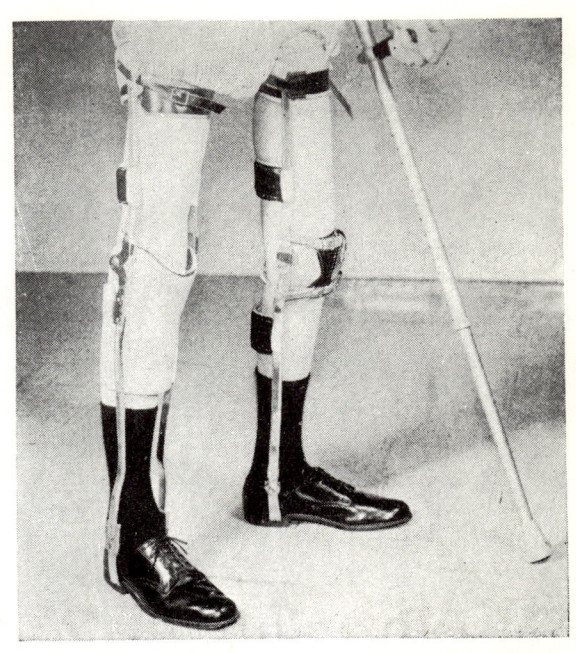

FIG. 1. This patient who has severe paralysis of both lower extremities is able to use a free-knee brace on his right leg because his hip extensors are graded Poor. On the left he requires a conventional locked-knee brace because he lacks all hip control in that extremity.

The third design is the UCLA hydraulic ankle control which offers graduated control of tibial advancement.

All three ankle units require a heavy-duty stirrup with an extended tongue to withstand the dorsiflexion forces as the body travels forward over the foot during the later portions of midstance and push-off.

The Knee Joint

The knee joint is set ¾-inch posterior to the midline of the leg so that the line of the patient's weight is anterior to the knee. As the patient's trunk and thigh move forward with momentum, the pressure on the thigh strap brings the proximal bar forward helping to keep the knee locked. The free-knee brace does not have to be made of special materials except for the heavy-duty, extended-tongue stirrup.

IV. Bracing for Patients with Traumatic Paraplegia

ELWIN EDBERG, B.S.

In bracing the lower extremities of patients with spinal cord injuries, potential problems other than motor paralysis must be defined.

Bracing needs vary according to the location and extent of the lesion. These needs must be identified by a thorough evaluation of the patient for muscular strength, sensation, and joint range. The muscle test should include the trunk and lower extremities. Patients who have incomplete lesions with scattered innervation of muscles in the lower extremities are also diagnosed as paraplegic, a situation sometimes overlooked by therapists. A thorough sensory evaluation to determine the areas of total or partial loss of sensation is essential. A range of motion test identifies areas of tightness or contracture. The patient's potential to use braces and the brace prescription are determined by the results of these tests in addition to the influence of other factors such as weight, age, sex, psychological outlook, cultural background, and home environment.

COMPLICATING FACTORS

Sensation

Total or partial sensory loss is overlooked many times in bracing a patient with paraplegia because of preoccupation with the motor loss.

Yet, walking may not be possible unless this sensory loss is considered. Because of his sensory deficit, a patient with traumatic paraplegia from a spinal cord injury is unable to walk without looking to see where his feet are placed, at least part of the time. In contrast, the patient whose paraplegia results from poliomyelitis can judge where his feet will land during walking without visual cues because his senses of touch and proprioception are intact (Fig. 1). This feeling of knowing where he is, and where he is going, allows him to use momentum gained from available muscular activity and to balance the trunk accordingly. Thus, the polio patient is able to walk more smoothly and with less muscular strength than the patient who is paraplegic from a spinal cord injury, even though the bracing requirements for both are similar.

This sensory deficit constantly threatens the patient with the possibility of developing pressure sores. These are avoided by proper bracing and teaching him to watch and care for his skin religiously. A simple reddened area is a first-degree pressure area. It will develop into a frank ulcer unless proper precautionary measures are taken to alleviate the cause of the pressure.

Bracing must be delayed until pressure sores are healed. Regardless of medication used, healing cannot take place as long as there is constant pressure. Common sites for these lesions are over the toes, heels, lateral malleoli, patellae, trochanters, and ischia. Braces, shoes, and tight trousers are sources of pressure.

Spasticity

If the patient has severe spasticity, it is futile to brace him for a goal of functional walking until the spasticity is relieved. Clinical experience has demonstrated that much of the spasticity in the extremities is aggravated by an associated contracture of the sensitive muscles. When this contracture is relieved by appropriate stretching techniques, there is often dramatic relief of the spasticity. The stretch reflex is not elicited as early nor as readily in the elongated muscles. For example, when patients with tight hamstrings finally achieve a straight-leg-raising range of 120 degrees, they no longer have spasticity to interfere with their functional activities (Fig. 2). When conservative procedures are not successful, surgery can relieve the spasticity to permit functional walking in carefully selected patients.

Patients with lesions distal to the first lumbar level will not have spasticity since the injury is in the area of the cauda equina and this constitutes a peripheral rather than a central nerve lesion.

Motivation

The patient's attitude toward walking is another problem frequently encountered. Almost all patients with paraplegia believe they

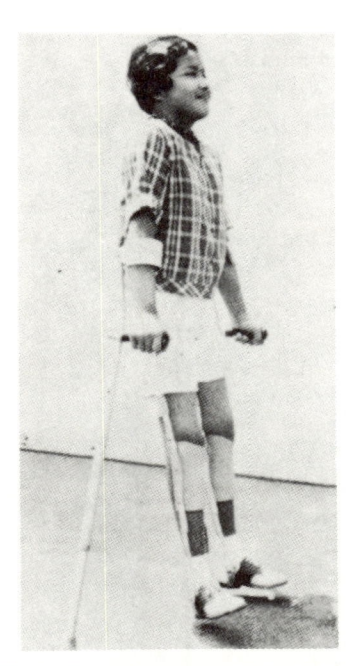

FIG. 1. A patient with complete paralysis of both lower extremities but who has intact sensation, such as this girl who had poliomyelitis, is able to execute a swing-through gait without looking at the ground.

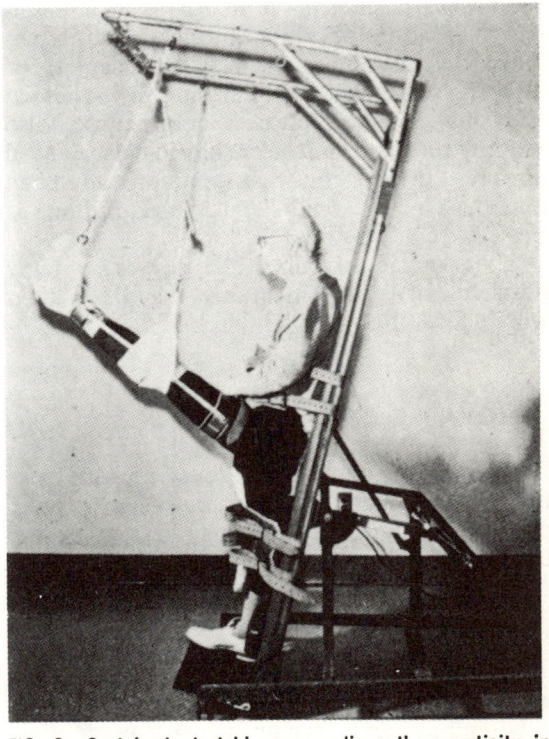

FIG. 2. Sustained stretching can relieve the spasticity in traumatic paraplegia. A range of 120 degrees of straight leg raising is necessary to permit functional activities.

will walk again. Their legs look all right, and because of the vague feelings of sensation which may change from day to day, and the evidence of motion through spasticity, they are certain that normal walking will someday be possible. Patients who have partial muscle innervation are usually reluctant to be braced. They believe that vigorous exercise will restore full strength. During this period it is important for the physical therapist to support the physician by emphasizing to the patient the importance of using the braces as a training measure so as to increase his use of the muscles which are now active. If function does return, the braces can be discarded and his physical condition will be better because of the activity during the intervening period.

Contracture

Contractures are a constant problem for paraplegics (Fig. 3). A hip flexion contracture must be stretched out before bracing is considered. Until the patient can fully extend his hips, he cannot balance in the upright position. Instead, he must compensate by putting all his weight on his crutches. Loss of this support as he lifts his crutches when attempting a swing-to or swing-through gait pattern makes his instability far worse particularly if he "jack-knifes" into acute flexion. Knee flexion and ankle plantar flexion contractures also prevent the patient from achieving a balanced posture. If these contractures are not stretched out, most of the time spent in gait training is wasted.

The struggle to walk in the face of so many obstacles gives little assurance that the patient will follow through after discharge.

MOVABLE SEGMENTS

For successful walking, four movable segments must be controlled by muscular activity, postural alignment, or bracing. These are the lumbar spine, hips, knees, and ankles (Fig. 4).

Lumbar Spine

Patients who follow through and become walkers are those whose trunk muscles (abdominals and erector spinae) grade Fair or better. This amount of muscular strength *can* stabilize the pelvis on the spine. Bracing is an impractical method of stabilizing the

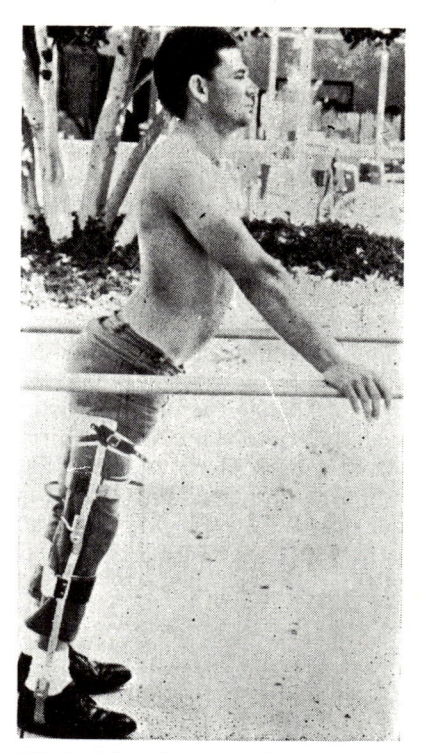

FIG. 3. This patient's hip flexion contractures must be stretched out before he can attain sufficient alignment stability for functional walking.

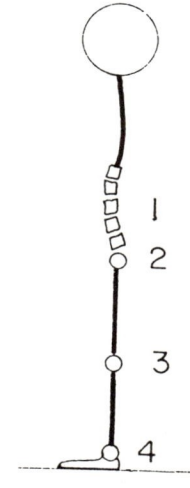

FIG. 4. The four moveable segments to be controlled in attaining functional ambulation in patients with traumatic paraplegia are (1) lumbar spine, (2) hips, (3) knees, and (4) ankles.

trunk because it makes walking much more difficult. When there is self-controlled trunk flexibility, the patient can alternately use flexion and extension of the trunk to assist in moving the pelvis with the lower extremities, resulting in a more efficient and smoother pattern of walking. Combined trunk rigidity and restriction of hip flexion hampers the essential activities of daily living such as wheel chair transfers and getting from the sitting to the upright position.

Knees

There are several ways of stabilizing the knee with a brace. One is the use of a conventional anterior knee control attached to the medial and lateral uprights of a long-leg brace. We have been experimenting with an anterior control strap placed either distal or proximal to the knee (Fig. 5). This eliminates increased pressure over the patella when the knee is flexed during sitting. Regardless of where the controls are placed, the limbs must be constantly watched for pressure areas. The knee joint of the brace can be locked either by drop locks or by bail locks. When bail locks are used there are no sharp points in the brace joint to cause rapid wearing of clothing over the area.

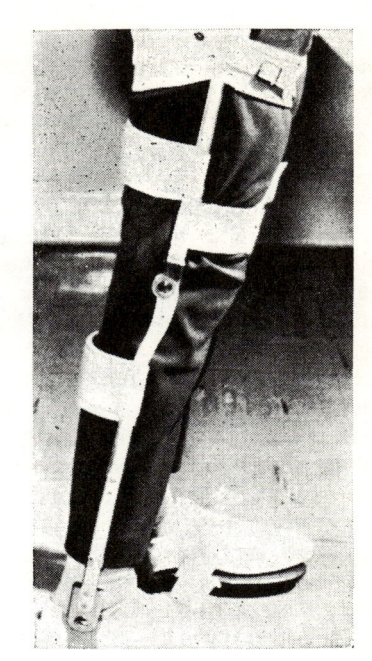

FIG. 5. To avoid increased patella pressure when sitting, the anterior control strap may be placed either proximal (as shown here) or distal to the knee.

Ankles

The ankles are best stabilized by means of an adjustable, locked joint on the brace (Fig. 6). Locking the joints in approximately 10 degrees of dorsiflexion assists the hips to extend on heel strike. The customary attachment of a brace stirrup riveted to the steel shank of the shoe is not sturdy enough to prevent bending. If the shank bends, much of the stabilization of the foot on the leg is lost. Motion from a weak shank has the same result as motion in the ankle. By building the stirrup and shank as a single unit of stainless steel, the necessary stability is gained.

Another feature of the brace should be a high-roll thigh band fitted 2 inches below the ischial tuberosity while the patient is standing erect. The thigh band is designed to give proximal brace stability on the femur without ischial weight bearing which would cause a pressure sore. The brace must be checked while the patient is standing, for if the patient is sitting or recumbent, the physical therapist is not able to ascertain where the thigh band will be when the brace is used functionally.

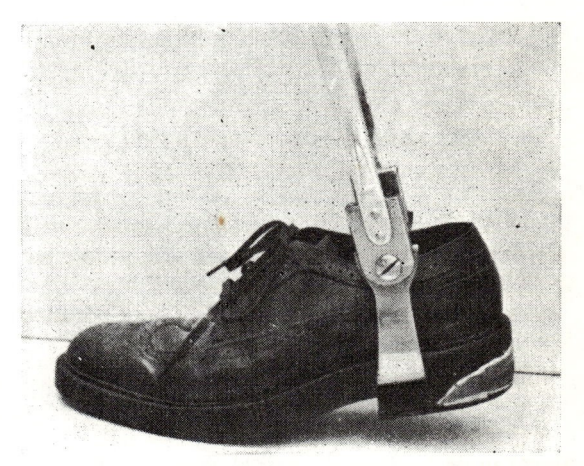

FIG. 6. The adjustable, locked ankle brace is locked in about 10 degrees of dorsiflexion. This assists hip extension at the time of heel strike. The force that is placed on the brace while it is held in a forward position demonstrates the locked ankle and the long-toe lever of the heavy-duty stirrup.

Hips

The hips are the only segment not stabilized by muscle or brace control. Stability is achieved by hyperextension of the hips and trunk. This allows the patient to lean into the anterior ligaments of the hips thus placing the pelvis forward of the center of gravity of the trunk. With the aid of crutches (axillary or forearm) he is able to maintain an erect position and walk for long periods of time. When the trunk muscles grade less than Fair, the patient can stand, but the amount of hyperextension needed is so great that the posture is not practical for walking. If the trunk muscles are Fair or better, the patient will be able to stand erect without the use of crutches (Fig. 7).

Controlling the hip joints through the use of a pelvic band is not efficient for several reasons:

1. The length of the lever arm of the lateral upright of the brace compared to that of the pelvic band is a ratio of eight to one. Hence, the stabilizing force of the pelvic band is poor unless tremendous pressure is exerted against the skin. The areas most susceptible to pressure are over the anterior-superior spine.

2. With or without hip locks, the patient has great difficulty applying and removing his braces independently if a pelvic band is attached.

3. A pelvic band limits the flexibility which a patient needs for activities such as stair climbing and curb jumping.

4. As much as 4 pounds of weight can be added to the braces by the band, thereby greatly limiting endurance for physical activity.

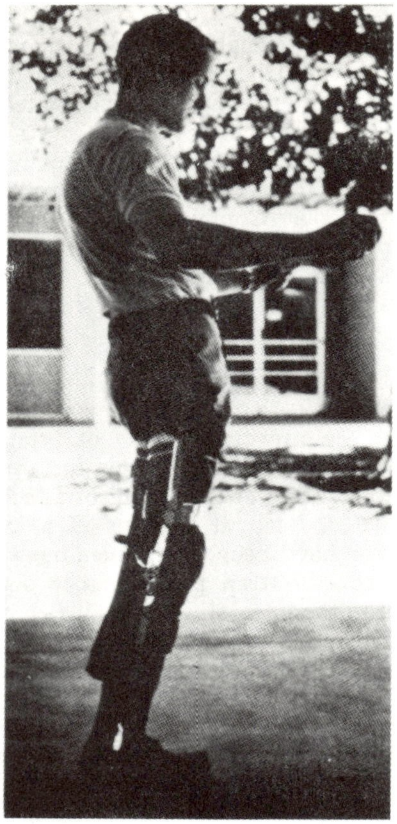

FIG. 7. This paraplegic patient has adequate trunk musculature and good range of hip hyperextension. He can stand erect without external support except for his long-leg braces which have been locked in dorsiflexion at the ankle.

SPECIAL BRACING PROBLEMS

The preceding discussion has related to the typical paraplegic patient who is braced to walk. There are other neurological conditions which present different bracing needs. The three most common ones are: Brown-Sequard syndrome, thoracic lesions, and low lumbar lesions.

Brown-Sequard Syndrome

When one side of the spinal cord is sectioned, a Brown-Sequard syndrome results. There is loss of motor control in one extremity with the sensation remaining intact. The other extremity presents the opposite picture, a loss of sensation but intact motor control.

Extremity with Sensory Loss. The majority of patients need a temporary short-leg brace for the extremity with sensory impairment to give added sensory input to the extremity. The brace should have an ankle upstop of 10 degrees and a downstop of 5 degrees with a dorsiflexion spring assist. The resulting resistance at the ankle joint is transmitted through the calf cuff as pressure against the gastrocsoleus area on weight acceptance. This pressure serves as a proprioceptive clue. On push-off, pressure is applied over the anterior surface of the tibia from the upstop. The short-leg brace also stabilizes the ankle and makes the patient feel more secure.

Extremity with Motor Loss. For stable walking the extremity with severe motor impairment and good sensation should be fitted initially with a long-leg brace having bilateral drop locks with ball-bearing catches at the knee.

Because sufficient return of muscular function often occurs, many of these patients progress to walking with an unlocked brace and eventually to using just a short-leg brace. The ankle joint should have no range in plantar flexion. This assists the patient to extend his hip on heel strike by the heel lever exaggerating the forward momentum of the thigh. There should be 10 degrees of motion in dorsiflexion at the ankle joint with a dorsi spring assist. The amount of tension on the spring will vary according to the weight of the foot and shoe, spasticity, and freedom of motion in the anatomical ankle joint.

Cauda Equina Lesions

Patients with cauda equina lesions who are free from the deformity can walk with short-leg braces even though the quadriceps test Poor minus, because all they need is ankle stability. A brace with an ankle upstop of 5 degrees in plantar flexion gives stability to the knee by action of the forefoot pushing the knee into extension on stance. Because full plantar flexion range is allowed, there should be a dorsi spring assist adjusted to lift the foot during swing to prevent the toe from dragging. Too much tension on the spring will create an added problem for the weak quadriceps during weight acceptance.

Thoracic Lesions

Patients with a lesion at T9 or above who have Zero or Poor abdominals have a very limited potential to walk even with long-leg braces. However, they may use them for standing at home. Those eligible for bracing in this group are usually young people who are extremely agile, highly motivated, and "fired up" for physical activity. Instead of using permanent braces, these patients do well with temporary posterior splints.

SUMMARY

Patients with pelvic control from residual trunk muscles which test Fair or better, and who have full hyperextension range in the hips, can attain functional ambulation with long-leg braces. These braces should have high-rolled thigh cuffs, locked-knee joints, anterior knee control straps, and adjustable ankle joints locked in approximately 10 degrees of dorsiflexion (Fig. 8). When the lesion involves L4 and lower, the patient can usually function well with short-leg braces, though they may need to start with long-leg braces if the quadriceps re-

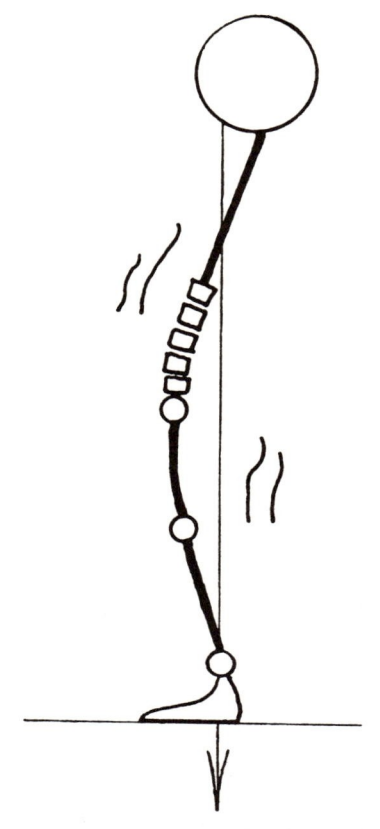

FIG. 8. Dynamic alignment for functional ambulation is attained through (1) trunk stability by active muscular control, (2) hip stability by a hyperextended posture, (3) knee stability with locked braces, and (4) ankle stability by adjustable joints locked in dorsiflexion.

gain their strength slowly. The patient with paraplegia who cannot stabilize his trunk over his pelvis (*i.e.,* lacks pelvic control) because of Poor abdominal and erector spinae muscles is not a candidate for functional ambulation.

Acknowledgement is extended to John Young, M.D., Craig Rehabilitation Center, Denver, and Shannon Stauffer, M.D., and Dale Fries, C.O., Rancho Los Amigos Hospital, for design of the brace described here.

SUGGESTED READING
1. Botek, Jean, Role of the Physical Therapist in Bracing. J. Amer. Phys. Ther. Ass., 32:236–243, May 1952.

V. Long-Leg Brace Design for Traumatic Paraplegia

DAVID HEIZER, C.O.

The customary braces that are fitted to the patient with traumatic paraplegia fail to permit him to achieve the goal of functional ambulation because they were originally designed to fit the more circumscribed problems of the poliomyelitis patient. Such braces do not satisfy the demands that are created by spasticity and lack of sensation. The dorsiflexion spring assist on conventional long-leg braces aggravates spasticity. To counter this problem, the braces have been made heavier and often a pelvic band or spinal brace has been attached to obtain hip and trunk control. As a result the braces became too heavy to be of functional use to the patient. We have never seen a patient with a pelvic band or spinal brace attachment on long-leg braces use such appliances for functional ambulation for any period of time.

Effective bracing for the spinal cord injury patient requires a new concept of joint alignment to attain adequate stability in the erect position, without the addition of a pelvic band or spinal brace, and without excessively heavy hardware.

We were encouraged by the success of locked-ankle braces developed at the Craig Rehabilitation Center in Denver. In a similar program, we have added our own modifications and incorporated a heavy-duty extended stirrup into the brace.[1] With the ankle in fixed dorsiflexion, the knee locked in full extension, with anterior knee flexion control pads, and a posterior thigh band, these braces allow the patient to balance his weight over his feet with the hips hyperextended. The center of gravity is kept posterior to the hip joint but anterior to the ankle joints to maintain the erect position. This eliminates the need for a pelvic band or a spinal brace.

THE STIRRUP

The heavy-duty stirrup consists of heat-treated 17-7 stainless steel which is almost impossible to bend. The tongue is lengthened so that it extends to the heads of the metatarsals—about 4 inches longer than the standard tongue on a stirrup (Fig. 1). In addition, it extends about 1 inch beyond the steel shank of the standard shoe. For additional strength, the tongue of the stirrup has also been widened about 1.5 inches over the standard design.

After the new stirrup is shaped and tempered, it is attached to the shoe and a new sole is put on over the entire device. The advantages of a heavy-duty extended stirrup are two-fold. It eliminates the customary breakage point where the stirrup is riveted to the steel shank, and it extends the toe lever. The average shank of the shoe breaks about mid-arch, whereas, with the extended tongue, the lever extends to the head of the metatarsals. This provides additional standing stability so that the paraplegic patient can stand in long-leg braces with extended hips, ankles locked in dorsiflexion, and without additional support of canes or crutches.

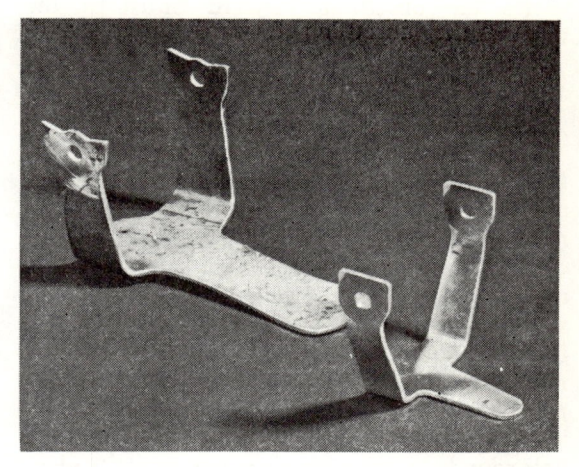

FIG. 1. The tongue of the heavy-duty extended stirrup (rear) has been lengthened so that it extends to the heads of the metatarsals. The older, lighter-weight stirrup (front) was subject to frequent breakage and had a shorter toe lever.

THE CUSHION HEEL

The second change in long-leg brace design to meet the needs of the paraplegic patient has been the addition of a foam rubber cushion in the heel to decrease the heel lever of the shoe (Fig. 2). Normally when the heel strikes the ground, the lever action throws the foot into plantar flexion. With the locked-ankle brace, this same force tends to thrust the braced extremity forward. This results in an awkward, jerky gait which also increases spasticity. The cushion heel, made of several layers of soft rubber, absorbs much of this force as the heel strikes the ground, providing a smoother gait.

THE ANKLE JOINT

An adjustable locked-ankle joint (Fig. 2) is used because the exact position of the ankle which allows the patient to balance in the upright position, varies with each individual. One-quarter-inch pins are placed under the screws in a double channel Klenzak-type joint and adjusted to lock the ankle in the proper position of dorsiflexion for the individual patient. The correct position is usually about 7 degrees of dorsiflexion. When first fitted the patient feels more secure with 10 to 12 degrees of dorsiflexion. As he gains control of the braces and learns to balance, he requires less and less dorsiflexion. An adjustable locking ankle joint, instead of the usual limited-ankle or

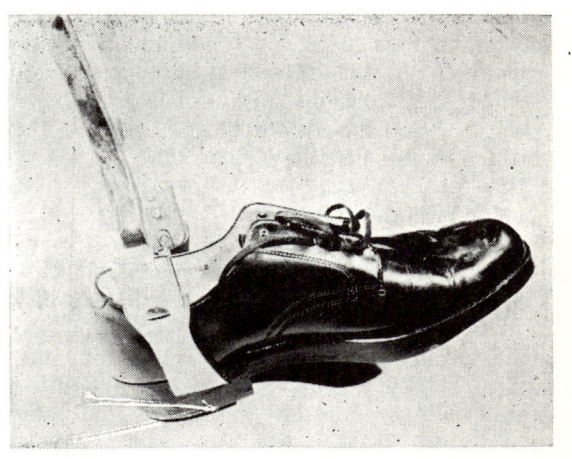

FIG. 2. A cushion heel, made of several layers of soft rubber, absorbs much of the force at heel strike, thereby providing a smoother gait. The ankle joint is an adjustable locked model so it can be fitted to the needs of the individual patient; this is usually locked in about 7 degrees of dorsiflexion.

arbitrarily locked-ankle joint, allows the therapist to adjust the brace as the patient progresses. The locked ankle transmits a greater stress to the stirrup during ambulation, thus the necessity for the heavy-duty stirrup.

As a result of these design changes, the paraplegic patient has a much more stable stance and gait. The locked dorsiflexion position of the ankle and the long toe lever assure a stable position of balance, and the cushion heel eliminates the unsettling forward thrust at the moment of heel strike.

THE BARS AND BANDS

The upright bars of the brace are made of Dural (2017T or 2024T aluminum alloy) and are slightly larger in width and thickness than the usual long-leg brace for flaccid paralysis. As used today, steel bars are much heavier, more fragile and become misshapen more readily. Therefore it is easier for the patient to bend his braces during normal use if they are made of steel. In the past, steel braces of light weight could be made by heating the steel and hammering it into a half-round shape which gave it strength. Today, it is difficult to find an orthotist who knows how to build a brace in this manner. Instead, a heavier, flat-bar stock is almost universally used and then ground down to the half-round shape. This makes the brace heavier and also weaker. An all-aluminum brace does not have the life expectancy at the joints that an old steel brace has; therefore, aluminum bars are available with steel inserts at the knee joint. This provides the durability of steel in the joint, but has the advantages of the lighter weight aluminum stock for the bars.

The material used for the bands is 0.090 inch aluminum. The bands should be wider than the usual long-leg brace bands so as to distribute the pressure more widely and prevent pressure sores. They must fit flat against the patient's leg to prevent skin folding or isolated pressure points. To avoid pinching the skin as the knee is flexed, the calf and midthigh bands are carefully placed so that they are not too close to the knee center of the brace. This means that the calf band should be approximately 3.5 inches below the knee center, the midthigh band approximately 4 inches above the knee center. This also permits the braces to be flexed beyond 90 degrees without putting pressure in the patient's popliteal area.

SUMMARY

The preferred brace for the traumatic paraplegic patient for functional ambulation (Fig. 3) consists of bilateral long-leg braces with an adjustable locked-ankle joint attached to a heavy-duty extended steel stirrup. The braces should also have posterior, molded leather, metal-reinforced thigh and calf bands, knee

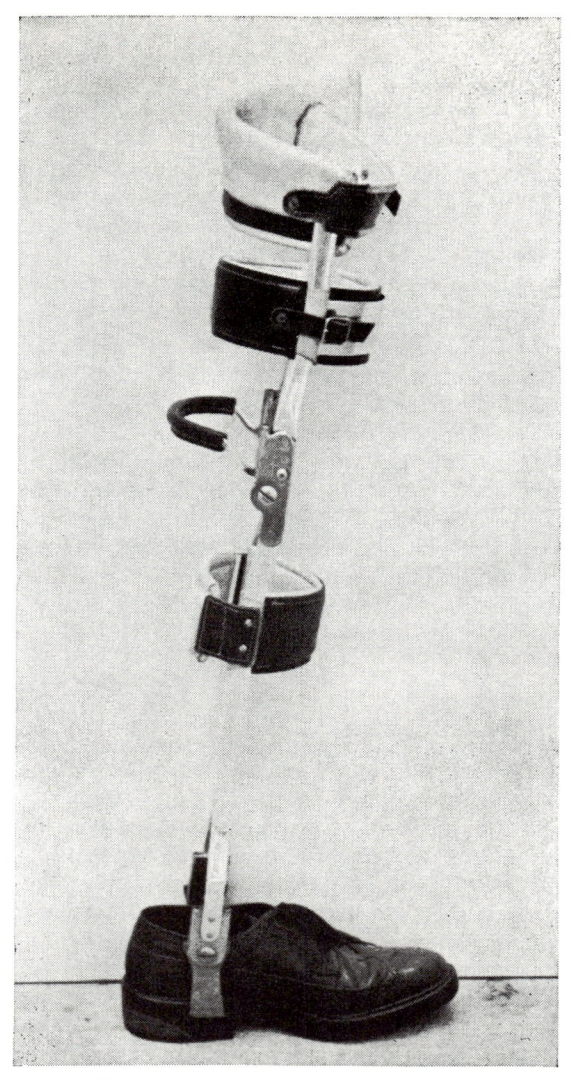

FIG. 3. The brace of choice for the traumatic paraplegia patient consists of double uprights, a high thigh rolled cuff, posterior molded thigh and calf bands, an adjustable locked-ankle joint, a heavy-duty stirrup, and a cushion heel. The brace illustrated shows two recommended modifications: a bail lock at the knee and anterior thigh and calf bands instead of an anterior knee control.

locks and an anterior knee flexion control pad. The shoes should be modified with a cushion heel of multilayered soft rubber.

Pelvic bands and spinal brace attachments are unnecessary items and have no place in the bracing of the traumatic paraplegic patient.

REFERENCE

1. Stauffer, E. Shannon, Elwin Edberg and Dale Fries. Functional Bracing for Ambulation in Paraplegia. In preparation.

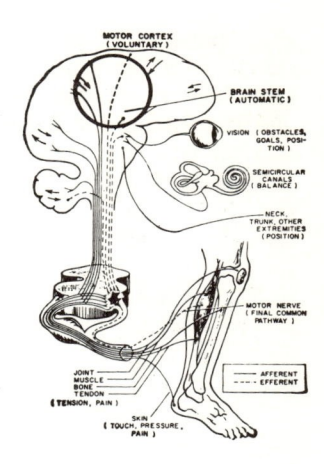

CONTROL DYSFUNCTION

I. Pathomechanics

JACQUELIN PERRY, M.D.

The inability to walk because cervical or thoracic spinal cord injuries have disrupted the motor and sensory message tracts is a relatively simple type of control dysfunction. Intellect, sensation and motor function are normal above the level of lesion. The separation between normal and disabled is not as obvious when the lesion is in the brain and intellect may also be impaired. This has been one of the areas of confusion in evaluating patients with cerebral palsy, strokes or brain trauma.

A second point of confusion is the fact that there are two levels of motor control within the brain (Fig. 1). Simple reflex synergies for

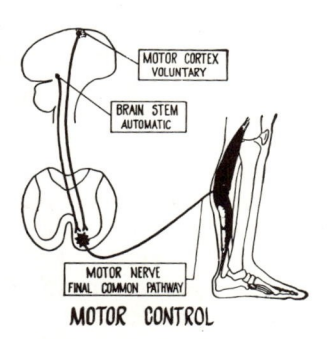

FIG. 1. Motor instructions are sent to the anterior horn cells from two areas within the brain: The cortex for selective motion and the brain stem for primitive patterns.

mass patterns of action reside within the residual primitive centers of the brain as representatives of simpler forms of life; selective and precise motor function originates in the cortical structures which are unique to man.[1]

The third aspect of the complexity of control dysfunction rests with the significance of sensation which is so readily overlooked. Persons learn to know exactly where their hand or foot is by the senses of stretch, pain and pressure within the joint structures, muscles, and skin (Fig. 2). These are related to the person's mental image of his body. When either the proprioceptive clues or the body image are distorted, subsequent motor performance which depended on this information is abnormal.

Another problem of motor function is a dependence on the mild, or normal, stretch reflex to provide protection when the extreme ranges of motion are approached. The sensitivity of the muscle to stretch encourages it to contract before the joint capsule or ligaments are stretched, and hence these tissues are protected from a damaging strain by prompt muscular action. The subtlety of response to stretch is lost when the selective motor control centers are damaged. As a result, there is an excessive response called spasticity. The final motor performance in the brain-damaged patient is a composite of impaired–to–absent selective control, reflex pattern activity and spasticity.

THE WALKING CYCLE AND CONTROL DYSFUNCTION

The relative values of selective versus patterned motion can be appreciated by a brief review of the walking cycle. For stereotyped movement the basic synergies of simultaneous hip, knee and ankle flexion or extension are utilized, as at the onset of the stance or swing phase. Selective control is needed, however, for further refinements of walking to accommodate for differences in limb length as the extremity position changes, and for the efficient utilization of momentum.

Stabilization of the extremity in the weight-accepting phase of stance consists of simultaneous hip, knee and ankle extension (Fig. 3). This corresponds to the primitive extensor reflex pattern. The pick-up phase of swing is also a reflex pattern, as there is simultaneous flexion of the hip, knee and ankle (Fig. 4). Thus, a

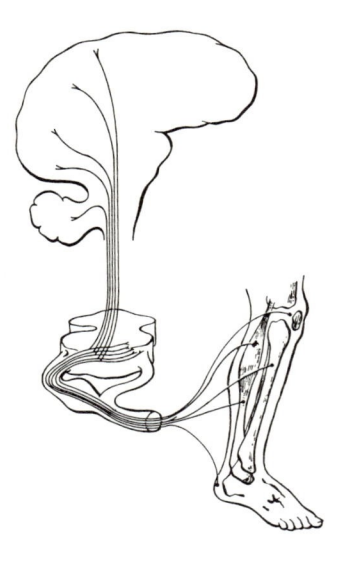

FIG. 2. Sensations of joint position, muscle tension, pain, and pressure, and so forth, are relayed to the cord and appropriate centers within the brain for assimilation and interpretation in order to guide the motor control centers as to proper motor instructions.

patient with only primitive patterns remaining, can walk by alternately using the mass flexor and extensor responses appropriately. On the other hand, normal walking requires maintenance of hip and ankle flexion as the knee is extended when the person reaches for the next step (Fig. 5). Gradual lessening of ankle extension, with continuous effort by the hip and knee extensors, is required as the trunk glides forward over the flat foot (Fig. 6). A marked increase in ankle plantar flexion is needed to push the person forward (Fig. 7). During the balance assist phase the ankle extensor muscles must be active at the same time the hip and knee flexors are contracting (Fig. 8).

In each of these phases of a normal gait cycle there is a mixture of flexion and extension patterns, or a variation in their strength. This requires selective co-ordination which is beyond the capability of the person with brain damage. As a result, these patients can be trained or equipped for safe and effective walking, but a normal pattern is not attainable unless there is complete neurological recovery.

REFERENCE

1. Krieg, Wendell J. S., Functional Neuroanatomy. First Edition. Blakiston Company, New York, 1945.

PATHOMECHANICS

POST HEEL STRIKE
WEIGHT ACCEPTANCE

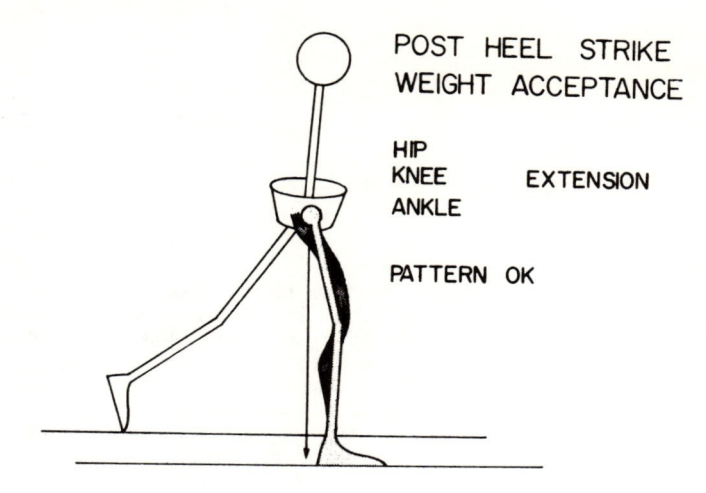

HIP
KNEE   EXTENSION
ANKLE

PATTERN OK

FIG. 3. A person can successfully support his weight with only the primitive extensor pattern since it corresponds to the normal simultaneous activity of the hip, knee, and ankle extensors as they stabilize the extremity for weight acceptance.

EARLY SWING
PICK UP

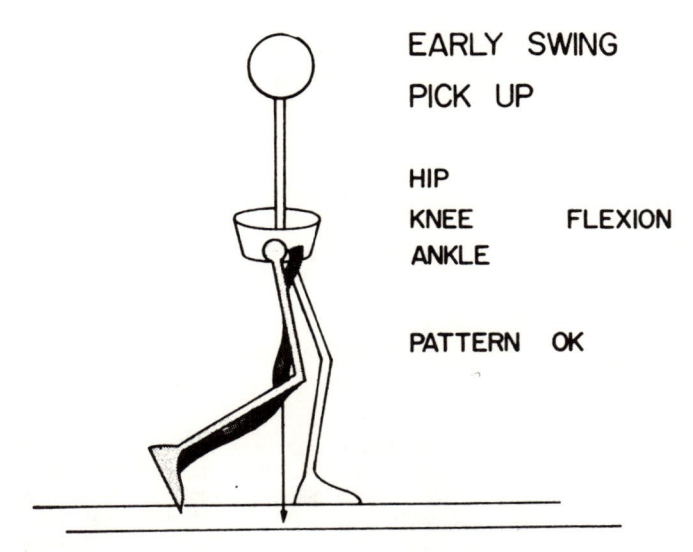

HIP
KNEE   FLEXION
ANKLE

PATTERN OK

FIG. 4. The patient who depends entirely on primitive patterns can take a step because this action corresponds to the normal simultaneous hip, knee, and ankle flexion of the pick-up task in early swing.

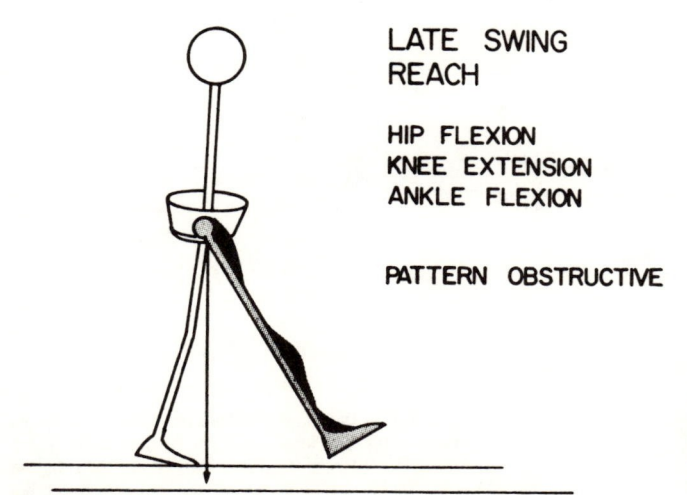

LATE SWING
REACH

HIP FLEXION
KNEE EXTENSION
ANKLE FLEXION

PATTERN OBSTRUCTIVE

FIG. 5. The patient dependent on primitive synergies for movement cannot take a step of normal length unless he falls forward as he is unable to extend his knee while keeping the hip and ankle flexed.

MID-STANCE
TRUNK GLIDE

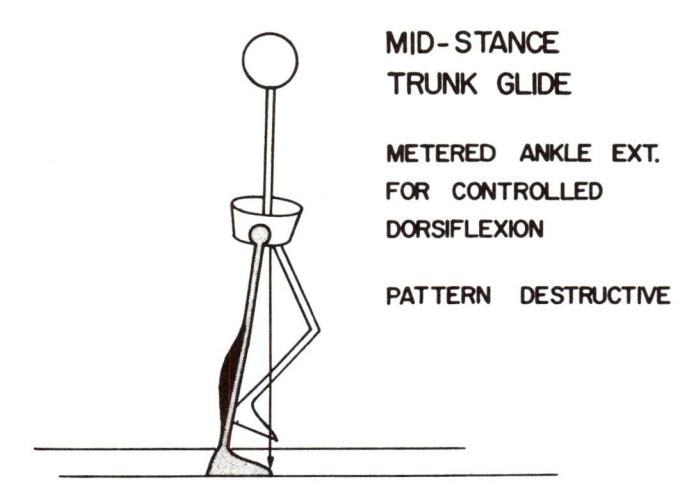

METERED ANKLE EXT.
FOR CONTROLLED
DORSIFLEXION

PATTERN DESTRUCTIVE

FIG. 6. The trunk normally glides forward over the flat foot by the gradual lessening of the plantar-flexion action of the soleus. Graduated control is not available to the patient who is dependent on primitive control patterns. To accommodate to the fixed ankle equinus which prevents his trunk balance over the foot, he quickly shifts his weight to the other foot. This results in shortening of the length of step taken by the normal leg in the hemiplegic patient.

PUSH

MAXIMUM ANKLE
EXTENSION (SEVEN MUSCLES)

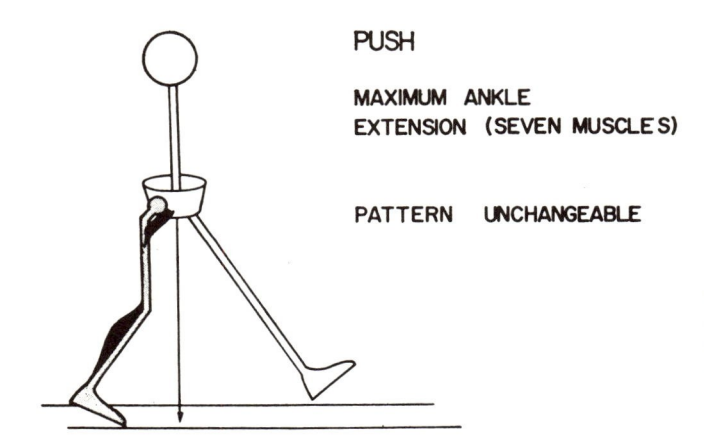

PATTERN UNCHANGEABLE

FIG. 7. Normal push force results from increased action of the plantar flexor muscles. The patient using primitive patterns cannot vary the activity of his muscles. The suggestion of push force that some patients evidence is due to the elasticity of the tense muscles or any contracture present.

END OF PUSH OFF
BALANCE ASSISTANCE

HIP EXTENDED
KNEE FLEXED
ANKLE EXTENDED

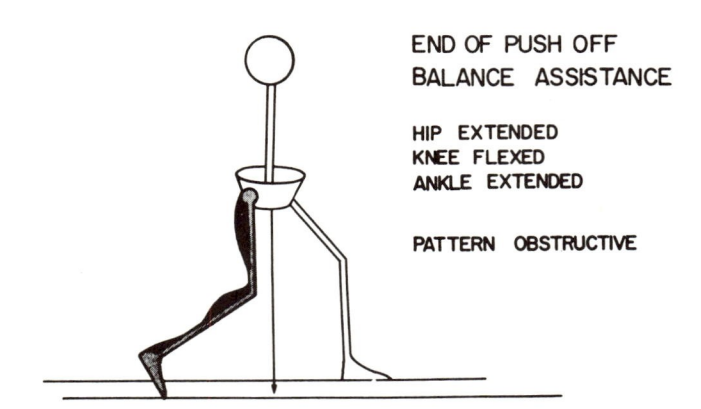

PATTERN OBSTRUCTIVE

FIG. 8. The limb that depends on primitive patterns cannot let the knee relax in flexion while there is active plantar flexion. Thus there will be no assistance with balance as the patient shifts his weight onto the other foot.

II. Control of Lower-Extremity Movement in Cerebral Palsy

SELECTIVE ACTION BRACING

VIRGINIA SCARAMUZZA GUESS, B.S.

THE PRINCIPAL LIMITING factors in the control of lower-extremity movement in cerebral palsy are defective voluntary muscular control and perceptual dysfunction. The manner in which the child receives and interprets sensory stimuli affects his motor performance. Children with cerebral palsy perform activities in gross patterns of movement. These patterns of movement can either be useful or they can interfere with function depending on the balance of their components.

The major components of the lower-extremity extension pattern are hip extension, knee extension, and ankle plantar flexion. The flexion pattern consists primarily of hip flexion, knee flexion, and ankle dorsiflexion. Children with cerebral palsy often have mixed patterns of movement as demonstrated in the typical extensor thrust which combines extension with adduction. Treatment goals are based on blocking the interfering, and developing the useful patterns of motion. The goals are attained through an integrated program of physical therapy, bracing, and surgery.

The traditional type of bracing for children with cerebral palsy is the bilateral, double-upright, long-leg brace with a pelvic band constructed with the intent of restricting movement (Fig. 1). These braces are heavy, cumbersome and definitely achieve their purpose of restricting motion. Such bracing provides a stable standing position but does not permit the amount of motion necessary for walking.

A more appropriate choice of brace design is that which restricts the interfering abnormal

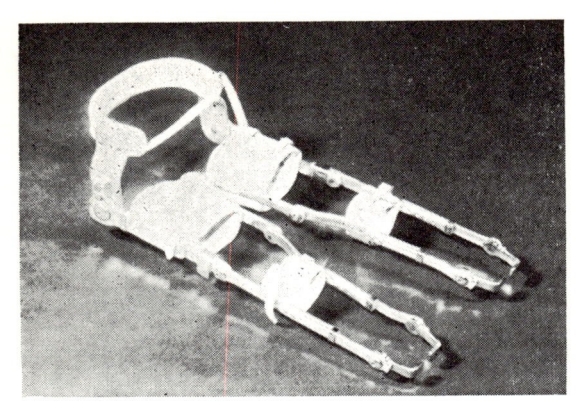

FIG. 1. Traditional bracing for patients with cerebral palsy consists of bilateral, double upright long-leg braces with a pelvic band.

motor patterns and yet still permits the child freedom of movement. These braces are used only until the child has developed control of his useful patterns of movement and are considered to be an adjunct to physical therapy.

PHYSICAL THERAPY

The first responsibility of the physical therapist is to observe and analyze the child's movements. The chronological sequence of motor development as observed in normal children has been universally used to assess the development of children with cerebral palsy. The child is observed while performing activities in the supine and prone positions, and when crawling, kneeling, standing, and walking. Of greatest importance is the level of development at which the child can perform with ease and also the level at which he has the most difficulty. It is at this next level—when the child is attempting to perform an activity with which he has difficulty—that an astute analysis of the movement is essential. The specific limiting factors that hinder the accomplishment of the activity must be determined.

The chronological sequence of development cannot be followed rigidly. Many normal children do not crawl before they walk. Furthermore, other factors such as neurological function and the presence of abnormal reflex patterns influence chronological development in children with cerebral palsy. As an example, a child with hemiplegia who is unable to crawl reciprocally may be able to walk in a reciprocal pattern (Fig. 2). He should not be detained from advancing to the next level which he is capable of performing. The child's ability to advance through this sequence depends on the maturation of the central nervous system, with resultant improvement in voluntary muscular control.

In analyzing the movement of children with cerebral palsy, the common terms used to describe problems in other diseases often are inappropriate. Terms such as "muscular weakness" or "lack of strength" may be meaningless in describing a child with defective voluntary muscular control. What is actually noted clinically is an overactivity of abnormal patterns of movement which limit useful activity. These patterns often result in deformity which further limits functional ability.

Because of the severe lack of voluntary muscular control, many children with cerebral palsy will not be able to walk. For these children, a treatment program, planned to develop control of the head, trunk, and upper extremity, is most practical. To walk, the child needs: (1) adequate head and trunk control to allow independent sitting balance (Fig. 3); and (2) adequate lower-extremity reciprocal motion with voluntary control of flexion and extension.

Following the analysis of movement, a coordinated program is planned to develop useful patterns of movement. While head and trunk control are necessary for walking, the most useful pattern of movement in the lower extremities is control of flexion and extension. Various techniques can be used to influence muscular activity. Once the abnormal patterns of movement have been identified, methods of blocking those patterns such as the use of reflex-inhibiting postures or prolonged application of ice may be used. Useful patterns of movement can be encouraged through various facilitation techniques such as cutaneous stimulation or passively imposed patterns of movement. These methods are included in the standard treatment of children with cerebral palsy.

However, these procedures are time-consuming and often are effective only during treatment.

Bracing with freedom of movement, except for selective control of unwanted movement, can increase the efficiency of treatment by prolonging the time the child's desired activity can be maintained. By the appropriate choice of brace design, unwanted movement can be limited while the child is permitted to move

BRACING IN CEREBRAL PALSY 65

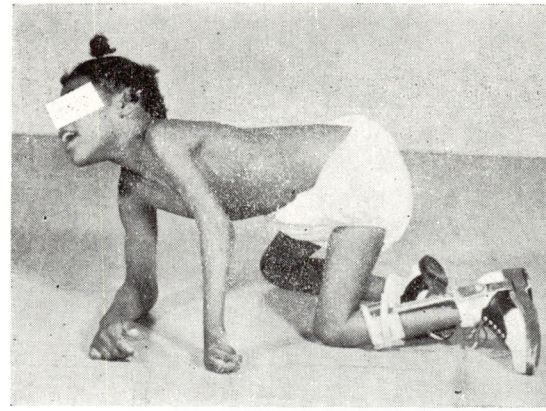

FIG. 2. Inability of this child to bear weight on her left arm (above) prevents her from crawling in a reciprocal pattern. The same child is able to walk with the support of one cane (right).

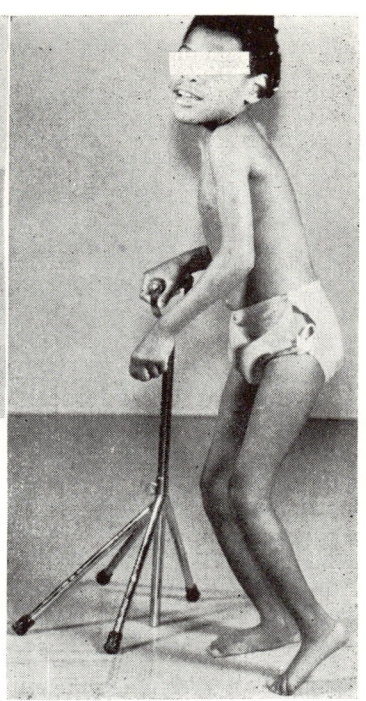

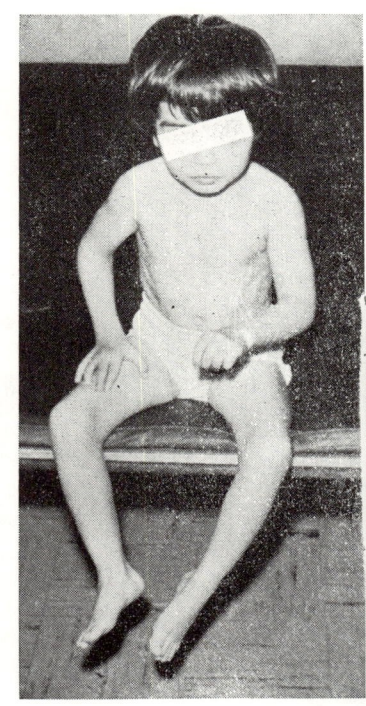

FIG. 3. Prerequisites for walking are independent sitting balance (left) and voluntary control of lower extremity flexion and extension (below).

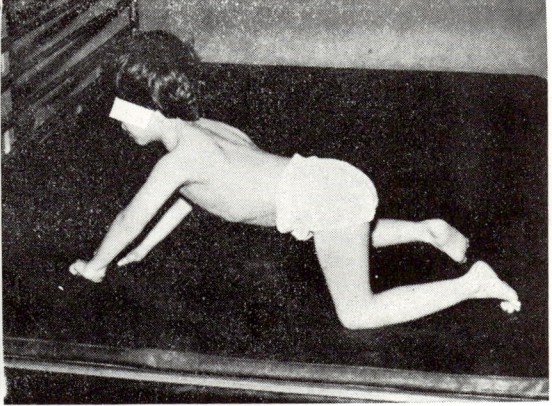

in useful patterns. This type of temporary selective action brace enables the child to practice desirable activity more hours in the day. Thus, he gains proficiency through prolonged repetition.

SELECTIVE ACTION BRACES

After a careful analysis of the patient's performance in which the major obstacles to effective walking or crawling have been identified, a brace is selected which will restrict this undesired motion with little or no limitation of other motions within the walking pattern. The hip, or the knee, or the ankle is braced individually as needed. Care is taken not to allow the brace to obstruct any useful motion.

Hip

One of the prerequisites for ambulation is lower-extremity reciprocation. Reciprocal motion in the child usually, but not always, begins in the crawling position. Spastic hip adductor muscles and an extensor thrust will interfere with the development of reciprocal crawling (Fig. 4, left).

Abduction Splint for Crawling. In order to block the unwanted adductor pattern of motion, an Ilfeld splint can be used (Fig. 4, center).[1] This is an abduction splint often prescribed by the physician to control dislocated or potentially dislocating hips. The splint consists of an adjustable spreader bar and two thigh cuffs. It prevents adduction, but allows some hip flexion and extension. Clinically, it has been observed that the splint is effective in blocking the spastic adductor muscles and allows the child to develop increased reciprocal motion (Fig. 4, right). Not only are the adductors blocked, but the abductor muscles of the hip are allowed to develop once the overpull of the adductors is decreased. In these splints, the child can crawl for several hours daily, practicing reciprocal crawling and exploring his environment.

Hip Action Brace for Walking. As the child moves on to higher developmental activities (such as the complex mechanics of walking in contrast to crawling), more freedom of motion in flexion, extension, and abduction is needed.

To control the spastic adductors and retain the other freedom, a hip action brace is used.[2] It consists of two leather thigh cuffs with hip joints attached to a pelvic band fitted below the anterior-superior spines. The hip joints are constructed to permit free abduction and to prevent adduction (Fig. 5). Just as the previously discussed abduction splint allowed the child to develop voluntary control of flexion and extension in the crawling position, this brace allows similar control to occur in the kneeling and standing positions. By eliminating the spreader bar, the hip action brace has the additional feature of permitting free flexion and extension of the hip which is necessary for reciprocal motion during walk-

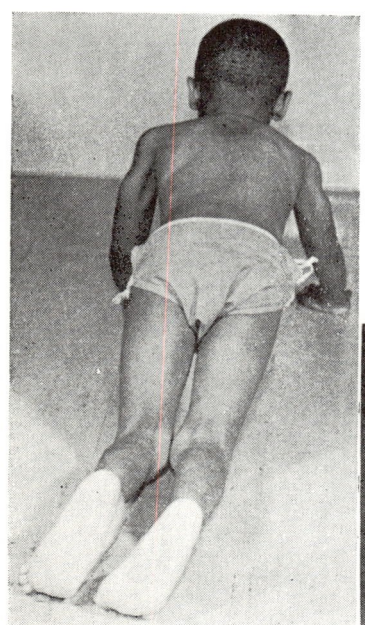

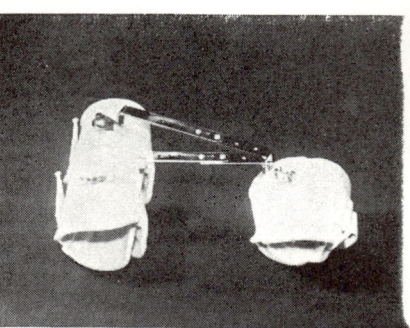

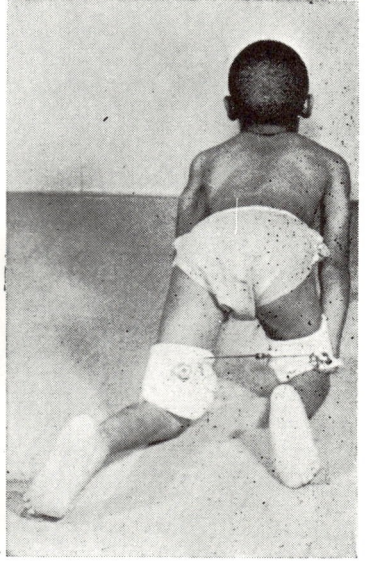

FIG. 4. Spastic hip adductor muscles (left) interfere with reciprocal movement. An Ilfeld abduction splint (center) with adjustable spreader bar and two thigh cuffs prevents hip adduction but allows flexion (right).

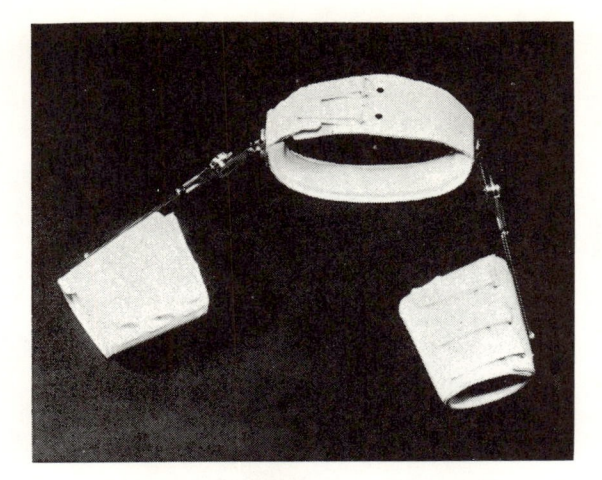

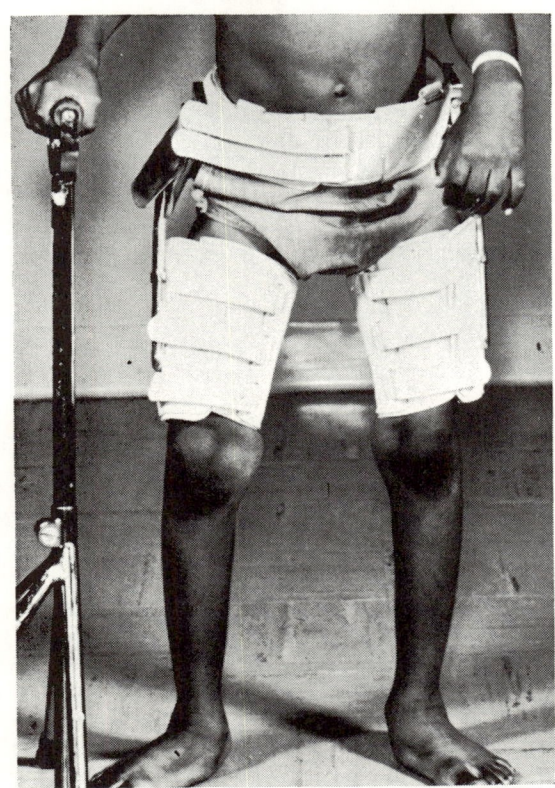

FIG. 5. The hip action brace (top) limits hip adduction and permits free abduction range of motion. It also permits an increased base of support (bottom).

Either the extension or flexion pattern may dominate lower-extremity movements in children with cerebral palsy; most commonly the flexion pattern is the stronger. Clinically, we have noted that when the hip action brace is first worn, the flexion pattern increases. That is, increased flexion occurs at the hips and the knees. This can be accounted for by the fact that muscles in the adductor group are also hip and knee flexors. Thus, when motion in one direction is restrained, tension of the muscles is concentrated in the other ranges. However, this increased flexion is a temporary situation as blocking of the adduction component of the flexion pattern permits the weaker extension pattern to be strengthened through increased weight bearing.

Twisters. Overactivity of the hip internal or external rotator muscles rarely is a problem in itself. Usually the rotation component is only part of a more complex pattern of movement. Twisters, which allow free flexion and extension, can be used to control either internal or external rotation when it exists as a single problem. It is often necessary to determine whether control of the rotation component alone will affect the total pattern. The twisters consist of four layers of steel helical weave encased in rubber tubing (Fig. 6). The cables are attached to a pelvic band and to a caliper in the shoe or to the lateral upright of a brace.

ing. This brace decreases the unwanted adductor activity, and at the same time provides stability at the hips. The design of the brace provides stability by widening the base of support in the kneeling and standing positions (Fig. 5).

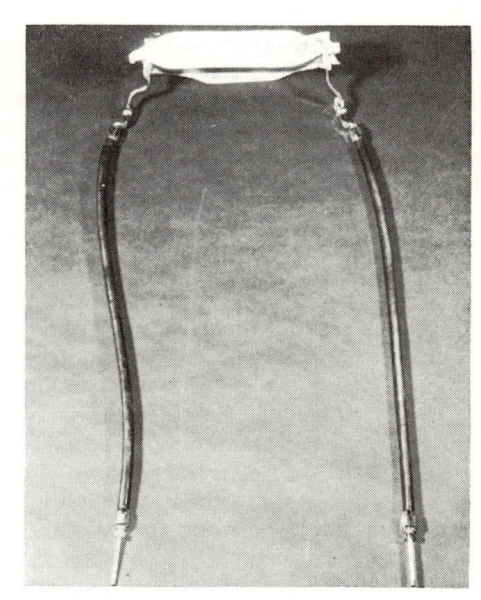

FIG. 6. Twisters may be used to control hip rotation.

Knee Cage for Extensor Pattern Assistance

Some cerebral-palsied children are unable to walk despite having reciprocal control of flexion and extension because they have inadequate strength of the extensor pattern. Clinically it has been noted that joint compression augments the extension pattern and can be facilitated through prolonged standing in a standing box or on a standing table.

A knee cage may be used as an additional training aid to develop an adequate extension pattern while walking (Fig. 7). The purpose of restricting knee flexion is not to provide knee stability, per se, but to support the child in extension so that he can develop his extensor pattern at the hip. Also, knee stability in itself is not usually the major problem in cerebral palsy.

If hip control and a secure placement of the foot on the floor can be obtained, the knee is stable. Once again, this temporary brace will permit the child to start walking sooner and to develop extension power as he performs the activity.

If the flexion pattern continues to be an overpowering force affecting the hip and knee, surgical release of the hip flexor muscles may be necessary to permit greater activity of the extension pattern.

Short Leg Brace for Ankle-Foot Stability

An analysis of the pattern of motion is essential if the factors that interfere with function are to be determined. In a child with hemiplegia, as an example, the common deterring factor to weight bearing is overactivity of the extension pattern. Two problems that result from excessive plantar flexion are marked equinus and inversion of the foot (either one or both place the foot in an unstable position) and extreme hyperextension of the knee on weight bearing. If the foot is not flat on the floor, but is held in equinus, the knee is forced into hyperextension as weight is taken on the extremity.

If the gastrocnemius-soleus spasticity is mild, a short-leg brace blocked at 90 degrees can be used to hold the ankle in a stable weight-bearing position. This brace not only puts the foot in a stable position, but also reduces the force that pulls the knee into hyperextension on weight bearing.

If, on the other hand, the problem is overactivity of the flexion pattern, then the problem will be excessive flexion of the hip, knee, and ankle. A short-leg brace with the ankle set in slight plantar flexion may reduce the flexion pattern by preventing dorsiflexion of the ankle.

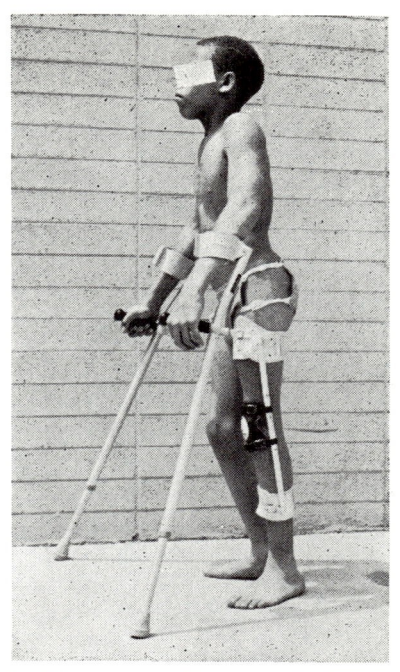

FIG. 7. A knee cage with an anterior knee control is used as a training aid to encourage the extensor pattern of motion.

RELATIONSHIP WITH SURGERY

The treatment program described consists of physical therapy, bracing, and surgery. Bracing not only serves as a valuable adjunct to physical therapy, but can also be used to predict the effectiveness of surgery. If bracing has adequately fulfilled its function of limiting unwanted motion and providing stability, then a surgical procedure may be considered to permanently decrease the force of the unwanted motion or to provide the needed stability. For example, a hip action brace can be used to ascertain whether the child's function is improved by blocking adduction at the hip. If the brace is advantageous, then a surgical procedure to transfer the adductor muscles posteriorly may be indicated to decrease the force of this pattern permanently. In this procedure, the adductor muscles that attach anteriorly are moved to the ischial tuberosity to decrease adductor power and supplement the extension pattern. With the decrease in adductor power, the hip abductor muscles usually improve in strength.

SUMMARY

Children with cerebral palsy usually have the longest treatment records and the shortest list of functional achievement. Perhaps it is time that physical therapists investigate new approaches to treating these children—methods that are practical and oriented to function. As therapists, we must be able to recognize when, and then be willing to admit that the child has reached a plateau in improvement. At this point, the child needs the equipment that is best suited to permit freedom of motion while reducing the interfering patterns of movement. Selective action bracing will permit him to be active at home and school until he is ready to advance to another developmental level. With routine follow-up care, the physical therapist can continually reassess his status. The use of this orthotic equipment makes efficient use of professional time and allows the child the freedom of movement needed for further development.

The equipment proposed for such use was: the abduction splint, the hip action brace, the knee cage, twisters, and the short-leg brace. They reflect the type of bracing that permits free movement and yet limits the overpowering spastic patterns. With these added dimensions of bracing that allow freedom of motion, the child can progress to more advanced patterns of movement. When the child learns to control these useful patterns without a brace, bracing should be discontinued.

REFERENCES

1. Ilfeld, F. W., The Management of Congenital Dislocation and Dysplasia of the Hip by Means of a Special Splint. J. Bone Joint Surg., 39A:99–109, 1957.
2. Garrett, A., M. Lister, and G. Bresnan, New Concepts in Bracing for Cerebral Palsy. J. Amer. Phys. Ther. Ass., 46:728–733, July 1966.

SUGGESTED READING

1. Holt, Kenneth S., Assessment of Cerebral Palsy. Lloyd Luke Ltd., London, 1965.

III. Bracing the Unstable Knee and Ankle in Hemiplegia

MARGARET INABA, B.S.

THE DIFFICULTIES the patient with hemiplegia has in stabilizing his knee during stance are of two types. The first problem is that of severe hyperextension or back knee. The second is that of the flexed or "buckling" knee.

THE HYPEREXTENDED KNEE

The hyperextended knee is caused by any of the following conditions: (1) weak quadriceps muscles, (2) impaired proprioception, and (3) severe spasticity or tightness in the plantar flexor muscles.

Weak quadriceps are often overlooked as a contributing factor. However, when a patient has weak extensors and is unable to control his knee in slight flexion he can compensate by locking it in hyperextension to gain stability.

Impaired proprioception also is overlooked as a possible cause for hyperextension. The patient attempts to compensate for his lack of sensation by snapping his knee into hyperextension. This gives him a sensory clue as to the position of his knee during walking.

Severe spasticity or tightness of the plantar flexors not only affect the ankle, but secondarily affect the knee. Plantar flexion causes the patient either to walk on his toes or to force his knee into hyperextension to get the foot flat on the ground as the trunk travels forward on the foot (Fig. 1).

Treatment

The most effective treatment for a hyperextended knee is a combination of quadriceps strengthening, short-leg bracing, gait training, and surgery. A short-leg brace is used as a mechanical support and also to provide a sensory clue to control hyperextension (Fig. 2). It is locked in slight dorsiflexion to prevent the knee from going into hyperextension. During forward progression, the force of the posterior cuff against the calf holds the knee in a neutral

BRACING PATIENTS WITH HEMIPLEGIA

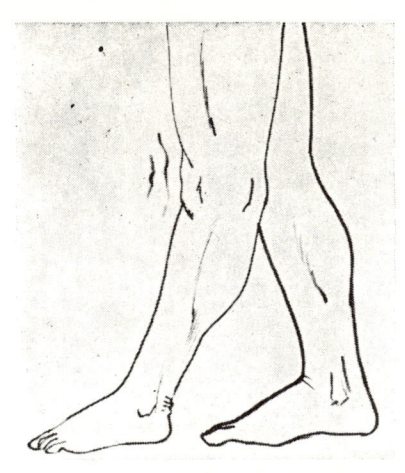

FIG. 1. Plantar flexion tightness causes the patient either to walk on his toes or in hyperextension to get the foot flat on the ground.

position by preventing the tibia from angling backward.

Spasticity of the calf muscles can be relieved temporarily by various facilitation techniques, but physical therapists have been unable to find a treatment which produces lasting reduction of spasticity, or correction of tightness which has occurred as a result of spasticity. When these problems continue to interfere with the patient's ability to stand or walk, surgery is indicated. Surgical releases or lengthenings of the posterior tibialis, toe flexors, and gastroc-soleus muscles, or phenol injections to the motor branches of the tibial nerve, have been used with good results.

THE UNSTABLE KNEE IN FLEXION

An unstable knee which buckles into flexion is not caused by weak knee extensor muscles alone (Fig. 3). The other possibilities are: weakness of the hip and ankle extensors; ankle dorsiflexion range of more than 90 degrees; impaired proprioception; and knee flexion contractures. If a patient is unable to compensate for quadriceps weakness by extending the thigh with the hip extensors and by extending the leg with the soleus, then his knee will "give" or "buckle" into flexion during forward progression (Fig. 3). The combined problems of weak quadriceps and plantar flexor muscles and an ankle dorsiflexion range of more than

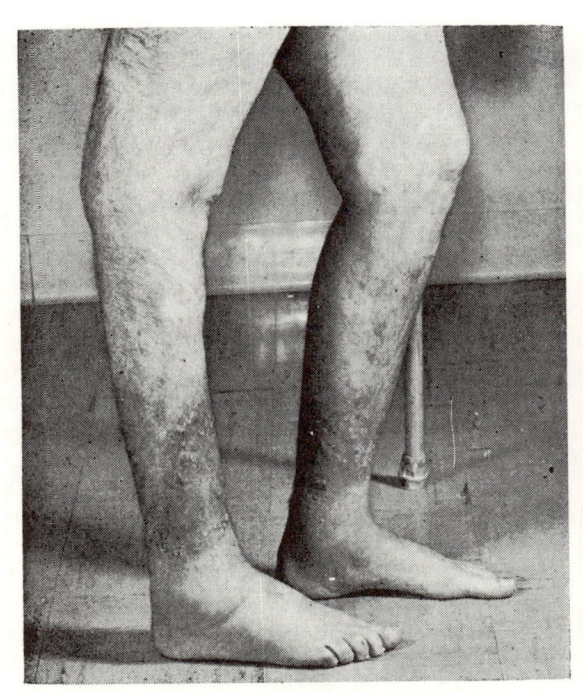

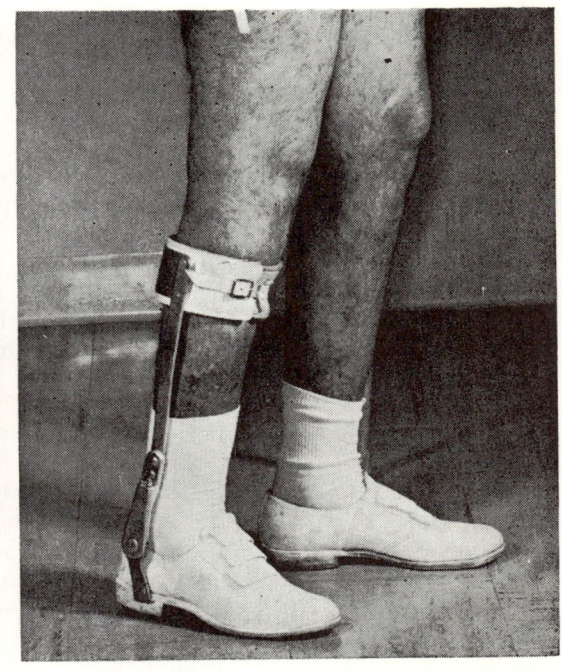

FIG. 2. The short leg brace is used as a mechanical support and to provide a sensory clue to control hyperextension. During forward progress the force of the posterior cuff against the calf holds the knee in neutral. The brace is locked in slight dorsiflexion.

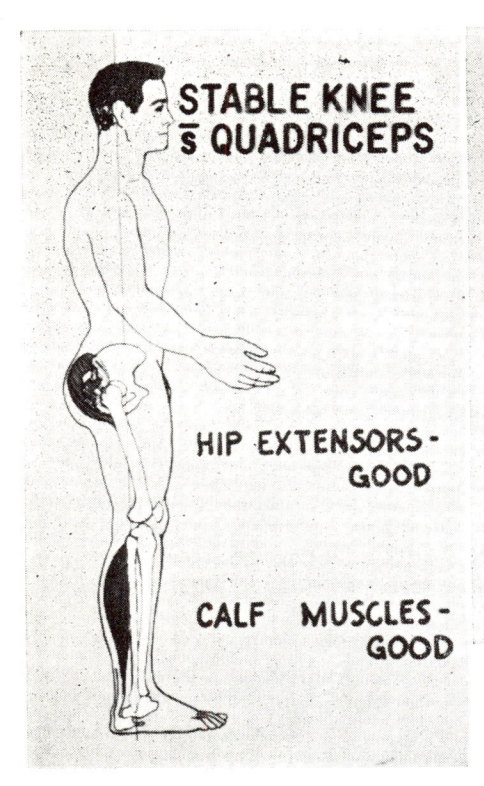

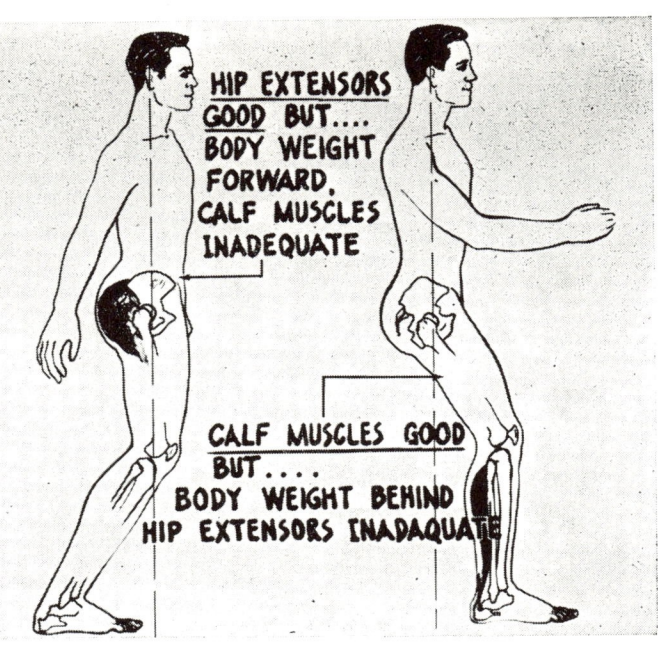

FIG. 3. When the quadriceps are absent (left) Good hip extensors and calf muscles can provide knee stability. Weak quadriceps and plantar flexor muscles and more than 90 degrees of ankle dorsiflexion are factors that cause knee collapse (above).

90 degrees allow the ankle to dorsiflex during weight bearing and, as a result, allow the knee to flex.

A patient with impaired proprioception or body image has difficulty realizing that his knee is too weak to bear weight. Therefore, he does not attempt to compensate for his lack of strength and puts most of his weight on the weak extremity which buckles into flexion.

Weak quadriceps muscles combined with a knee flexion contracture force the knee to flex during weight bearing. Much more strength is required to walk with a flexed knee than with a knee that can extend fully.

Treatment

Treatment for instability in flexion is a combination of (1) strengthening, (2) stretching and positioning to correct knee flexion contractures, (3) positioning to develop a functional contracture in the ankle plantar flexor muscles, (4) adjustment of the short leg brace to 90 degrees or in slight plantar flexion, and (5) gait training.

Progressive resistive exercise to reinforce the extension synergy or mass extension pattern is given in the supine or standing position. If the patient has selective control, which is the ability to stabilize one joint while selectively moving another, progressive resistive exercises are given to the selective movements rather than to the mass patterns.

A patient with a knee flexion contracture is placed on a static stretch by applying weights behind the upper part of his tibia, as well as at his ankle, to encourage a gliding motion at the knee (Fig. 4). If the weight behind the upper part of the tibia is omitted, the weight at the ankle jams the tibia against the femur and causes pain at the anterior margin of the joint. A static stretch for one-half hour once or twice a day is not enough to reduce the contracture. A positioning program must supplement the stretching program.

Prone positioning on a guerney is effective for the more alert and co-operative patient. However, if the patient is confused, staying prone during the day for several hours at a time only seems to increase his mental disorientation. Also, if he has a painful shoulder, it it difficult to make him comfortable in this

BRACING PATIENTS WITH HEMIPLEGIA

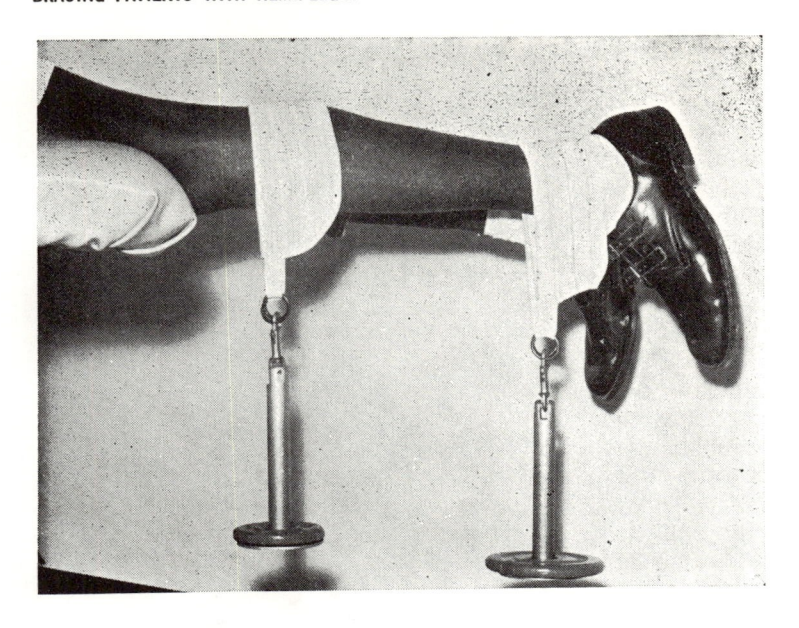

FIG. 4. Weights are hung over the upper portion of the tibia and at the ankle when the patient is prone with his leg over the end of a plinth. This places a static stretch on a knee flexion contracture with forward gliding of the tibia.

position. The prone position is effective for patients who can tolerate it, especially if they lie prone intermittently both day and night.

Maximum knee extension range can be achieved by having the patient wear a long-leg knee cage or plaster splint for as much of a twenty-four-hour period as possible. However, if the patient has severe spasticity, these two devices may cause pressure areas on the skin.

Prolonged standing in a Stand-alone ® walker (Fig. 5), on the tilt table, or in parallel bars with the knee in extension are very effective methods of positioning. Standing allows the patient to view his surroundings in the normal perspective, and weight bearing stimulates the function of the mass extension pattern. This pattern also helps to reduce a knee flexion contracture. If the contracture is severe, the treatment approach includes not only stretching and positioning, but also surgery and progressive casting.

Control of the Unstable Knee by Positioning the Ankle

A short leg brace locked at 90 degrees is used if the patient has an unstable knee which buckles into flexion, weak plantar flexor muscles, and more than 90 degrees of range in dorsiflexion. This brace encourages the development of a functional plantar flexion contracture which acts as a checkrein on the knee. When the ankle is locked at 90 degrees and

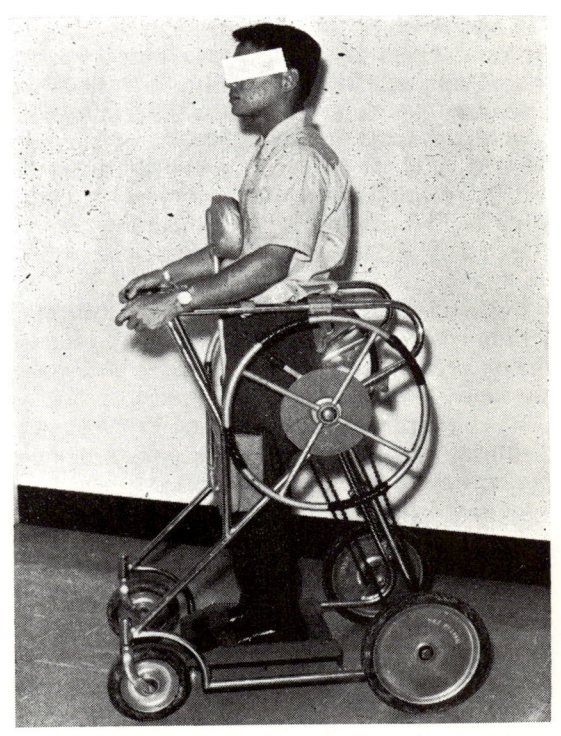

FIG. 5. Prolonged standing with the knee in extension is an effective method of positioning.

the hip extensors extend the thigh, the knee cannot buckle into flexion.

A short-leg brace, locked at 90 degrees or in slight plantar flexion, is used also as a sensory cue to prevent the knee from buckling into flexion. The locked ankle joint which prevents dorsiflexion causes cuff pressure against the anterior part of the tibia (Fig. 6). This stimulus causes the patient to contract the quadriceps and hip extensors (to pull away from the brace) thereby gaining the desired knee stability.

If the patient has inadequate strength in the hip extensor muscles, or has such impaired proprioception that he cannot stabilize the knee with the help of a short-leg brace, a knee cage is used as a temporary training device (Fig. 7). This device is needed only until the patient develops more awareness of his affected extremity, or until the hip extensors are of sufficient strength to extend the knee.

Long-Leg Braces

The patient with hemiplegia needs hip extensor strength to use either a long-leg or a short-leg brace. To walk with a long-leg brace he needs enough hip extension control to counteract spasticity or tightness of the hip flexors, *i.e.*, to stabilize the trunk over the weight-bearing extremity. Yet, when there is this much hip control present, there is adequate thigh stability for a short-leg brace to stabilize the knee.

Since the unstable knee can be controlled with a short-leg brace, this is the brace of choice. It conserves the patient's energy because it is lighter and permits the knee to flex during the swing phase of gait. Patients with little use of one upper extremity and even those who are mentally confused can easily put on a short-leg brace without assistance.

THE UNSTABLE ANKLE

The indications for bracing the ankle in patients with hemiplegia are: drop foot, equinovarus, and impaired proprioception. The causes of drop foot are: (1) weak dorsiflexor muscles, especially the extensor digitorum longus, (2) dorsiflexors which function late in the forward swing phase, and (3) spastic or tight plantar flexors.

Treatment includes resistive exercise, gait training, and adjustment of the short-leg brace to a 90 degree downstop.

If ankle dorsiflexion occurs in a mass flexion

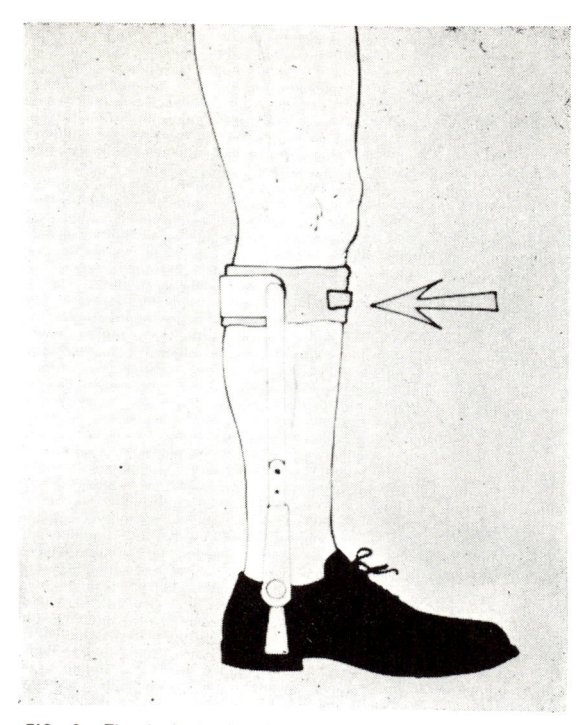

FIG. 6. The locked-ankle joint which prevents dorsiflexion, causes cuff pressure against the anterior part of the tibia. This stimulus causes the patient to contract the quadriceps and hip extensors thus preventing the knee from buckling into flexion.

pattern, resistance is given to the total pattern to reinforce the tibialis anterior. Resistance to hip flexion during walking stimulates ankle dorsiflexion. However, if the patient has selective control, the selective motion is strengthened.

When the patient has a simple drop foot with no plantar flexion spasticity, a coil spring brace can be used. If slight plantar flexion spasticity or tightness is present, a Klenzak-type brace with a dorsiflexion spring-assist is indicated. If plantar flexion spasticity or tightness is more severe, the dorsi assist will not be strong enough to dorsiflex the ankle and will aggravate the spasticity. In this case, a brace with a 90-degree downstop is indicated.

Equinovarus is caused by an overactive tibialis anterior, weak evertors and spasticity in the toe flexors, tibialis posterior and gastrocsoleus muscles. Treatment includes bracing and sometimes surgery. A sturdy brace with double uprights is needed to control the equinovarus. The coil spring brace is not strong enough to provide ankle stability. If the pa-

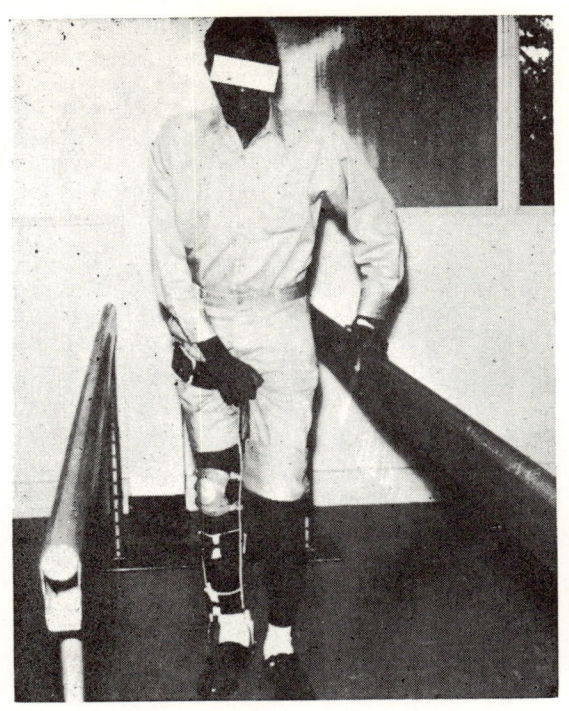

FIG. 7. A knee cage is used as a temporary training device for patients with weak hip extensor muscles or markedly impaired proprioception.

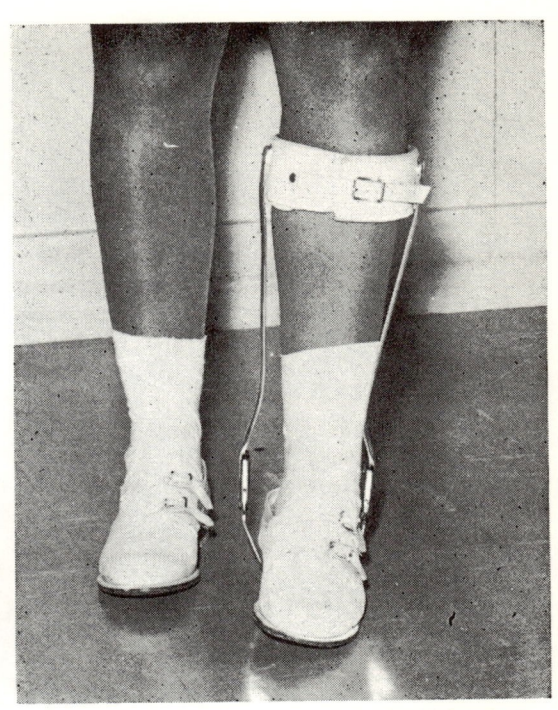

FIG. 8. A severe equinovarus uncontrolled by bracing.

tient's deformity is so severe that it cannot be controlled by the brace (Fig. 8), surgery is considered. If the tibialis anterior is contributing to the varus, the surgeon divides the tendon and transfers half of it laterally to the third cuneiform. If the toe flexors, tibialis posterior, and gastroc-soleus muscles are producing a deformity, the surgeon releases or lengthens these muscles, or sometimes injects the nerve with phenol.

Occasionally a patient with hemiplegia who has good motor control but impaired proprioception, moves his foot back and forth into inversion and eversion during forward swing. This extraneous movement causes him to land on the lateral border of his foot. A short-leg brace enables him to bear weight on the plantar surface of the foot, thus making walking a safe activity.

SUMMARY

In summary, a short-leg brace is a useful adjunct for the patient with hemiplegia who has an unstable knee, drop foot, equinovarus, or impaired proprioception.

IV. Short-Leg Brace Design for Hemiplegia

DAVID HEIZER, C.O.

The patient with hemiplegia uses a short-leg brace to stimulate proprioception, to provide ankle control, to prevent plantar flexion contractures of the ankle, and to assist dorsiflexion.

Three basic brace designs are available. These are: (1) the coil spring, toe pick-up brace, (2) the limited-motion brace, and (3) the double adjustable ankle joint brace.

THE COIL SPRING BRACE

The coil spring, toe pick-up brace is the simplest of the short-leg braces (Fig. 1). It is lightweight, easily adjusted, and cosmetically acceptable. This brace does not offer knee stability because it cannot be limited in either plantar flexion or dorsiflexion. Neither does it offer ankle stability because of the lightweight material used in its construction. The

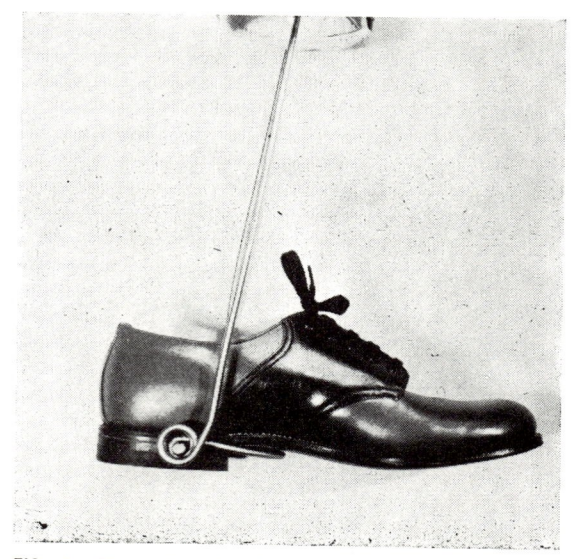

FIG. 1. The coil spring brace is lightweight and easily adjusted but its only value is as a dorsiflexion assist for a flaccid drop foot.

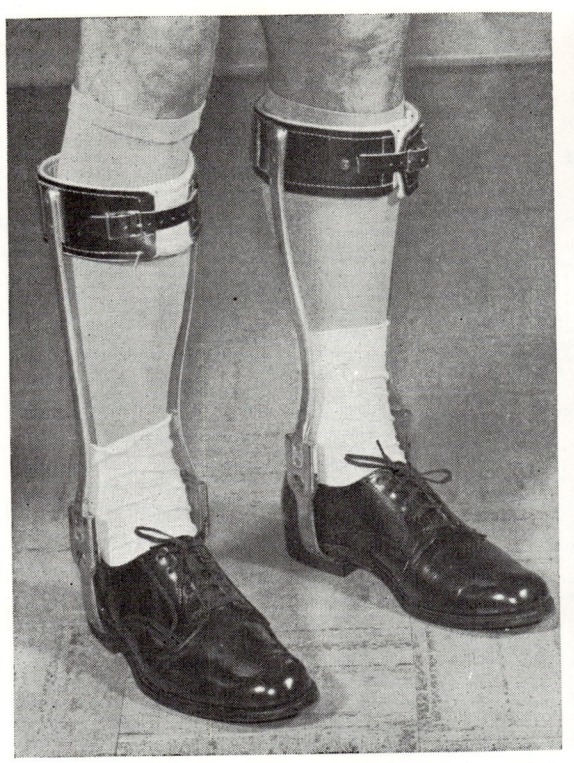

FIG. 2. The preferable brace for the hemiplegic patient with instability, deformity or spasticity is the double adjustable ankle brace. This particular brace is the Becker-type in which the channels are anterior and posterior to the uprights.

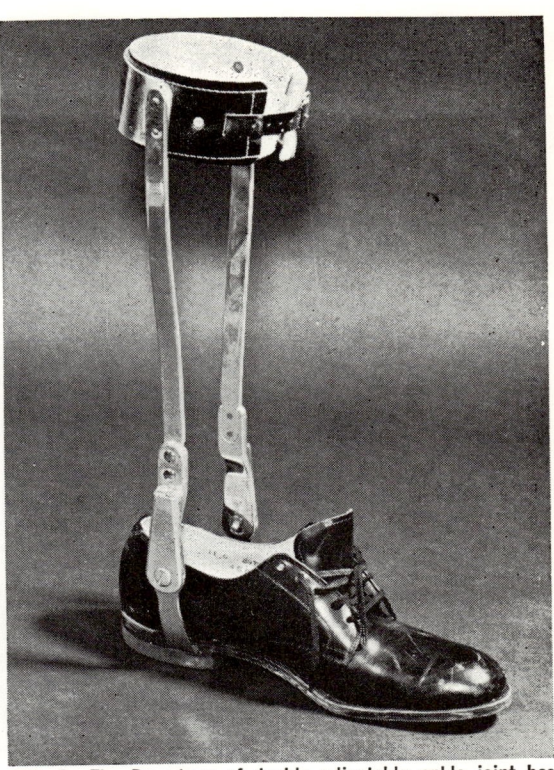

FIG. 3. The Pope-type of double adjustable ankle joint has the channels placed lateral to the uprights.

brace is made of ⅛-inch stainless steel spring wire with four coils at the shoe. The amount of dorsiflexion assistance provided is adjusted by changing the angle of the last coil on both sides of the shoe.

All this brace does is pick up a flaccid drop-foot when there is no calf muscle spasticity.

THE LIMITED MOTION BRACE

The limited motion brace is made of aluminum.

The stops are ground to allow range in 10 degrees of dorsiflexion and 10 degrees of plantar flexion. It is used only for proprioception problems. The weight of the brace during the swing phase, and the impact of the brace against the leg at weight-acceptance, offers the patient sensory clues and, therefore, provides him with a safer and smoother gait.

THE DOUBLE ADJUSTABLE ANKLE BRACE

A brace with a double adjustable ankle joint is the brace of choice for the patient with hemiplegia (Fig. 2). It provides limited motion in any range of ankle motion desired and can include a dorsiflexion spring assist. The front springs are removed and ¼-inch pins are substituted; ⅛-inch pins are put inside the back springs. By turning set screws in the joint, the motion can be limited as needed and the patient can still obtain dorsiflexion assistance. Dorsiflexion assists should not be used if spasticity or clonus are present. To give the individual patient knee stability, the double adjustable brace can be locked in any degree of dorsiflexion and plantar flexion.

To lock the brace, the front and back springs are removed and replaced with ¼-inch pins. The set screws are tightened until the joint is locked.

There are two double adjustable brace

joints currently available. The Pope brace has an inset built into the bars (Fig. 3). This type of joint provides active dorsiflexion assist and about 5 degrees of range of motion. The bulk and limited adjustability are disadvantages with the hemiplegic patient.

The Becker is a smaller brace unit (Fig. 2). It permits a full range of motion and has a dorsiflexion assist although its dorsiflexion spring is extremely stiff. The springs are short and very strong, causing them to load quickly. This causes very rapid dorsiflexion.

However, substitution of a lighter spring solves the problem. Patients seem to accept this type of brace joint over the first because it can be made to be more acceptable cosmetically. The joint can be placed closer to the malleolus (⅜ to ¼ inches away) in contrast to the ¾-inch distance for the other adjustable design. The bars are shaped so they fit ½ inch or less from the leg. The calf band is placed 1 inch below the head of the fibula to avoid perssure on the common peroneal nerve.

FIG. 4. An arch support is used to hold the foot out of valgus as it gives more correction than a T-strap. The tear-drop-shaped arch support (left) is made from hard sponge rubber. The arch support is placed in the shoe (right) with the high point about one-third the distance between the calcaneus and the head of the first metatarsal.

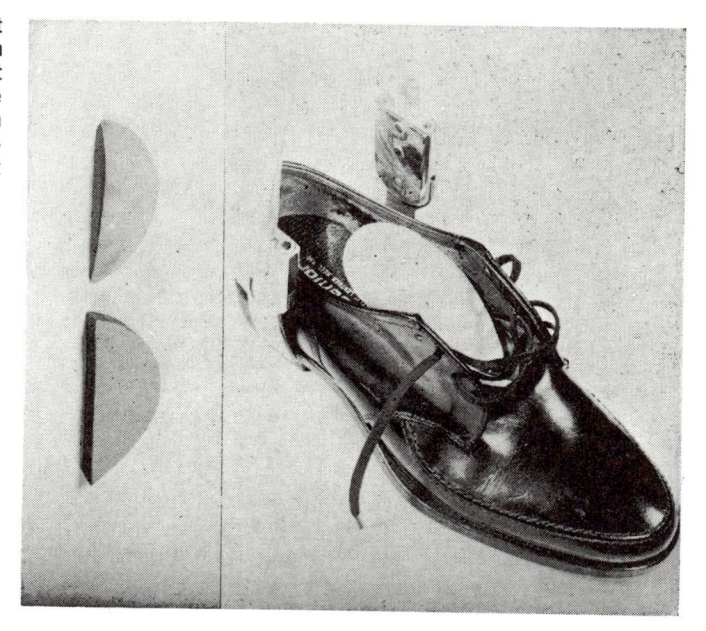

FIG. 5. A wedge may be used on the lateral border of the heel of the shoe to correct a varus.

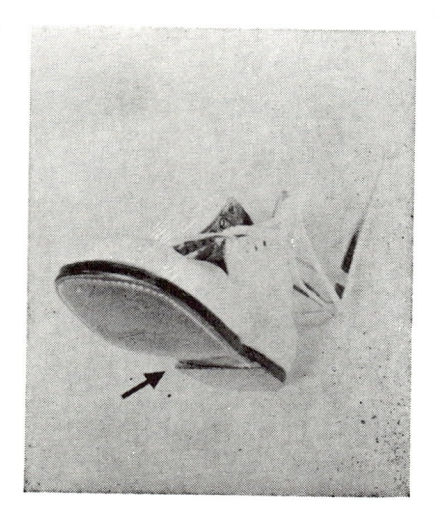

BRACE DESIGN FOR HEMIPLEGIA

For more difficult problems in knee extension, a pretibial shell is added to the short-leg brace with an adjustable ankle joint. The ankle then is locked in slight plantar flexion to hold the knee in extension. A heavy-duty extended stirrup is used with this brace which is made of 17-7 tempered stainless steel. The stirrup extension lengthens the toe lever so there is more force to extend the knee.

Valgus

When the foot goes into valgus, a high longitudinal arch support is inserted in the shoe (Fig. 4). This is made of firm sponge rubber, shaped to resemble half a teardrop. It is glued into the shoe with the high point at about one-third the distance between the calcaneous and the head of the first metatarsal. This pad gives more correction than a T-strap. A T-strap does not really correct a valgus condition, it just pushes against the medial malleolus.

Varus

When the patient's foot is in varus, a wedge is placed between the stirrup and the shoe on the lateral border of the heel (Fig. 5). This tips the foot out of varus into a neutral plane. Tibial torsion is built into the brace by bending the lateral brace bar back and the medial bar forward an equal distance. The bars are then twisted laterally until they are square in all planes. This rotates the foot outward to its proper relationship with the tibia.

The Shoe

Thus far, little has been said about shoes used in conjunction with leg braces, yet the shoe is the foundation for every brace. The more limitations that are placed on the ankle joint of the brace, the better the shoe must be and the stronger the shank. Even the coil spring toe pickup brace makes it necessary to have a steel shank in the shoe. Without the shank, a ridge appears on the inside of

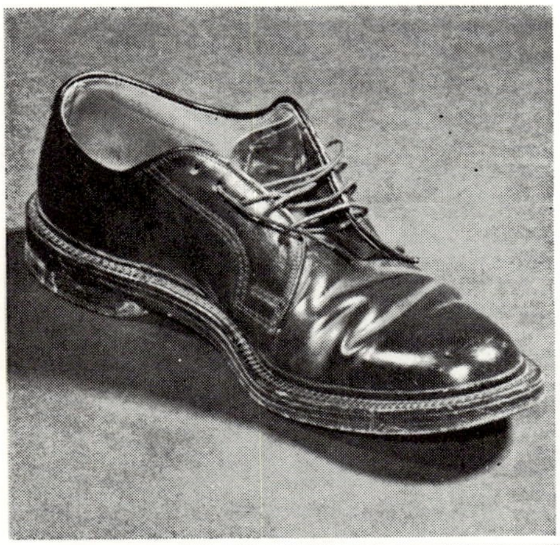

FIG. 6. The Blucher-style shoe (left) is preferred when the patient requires a brace. The Balmoral-style shoe (below) has a "V" opening which makes it harder to put on.

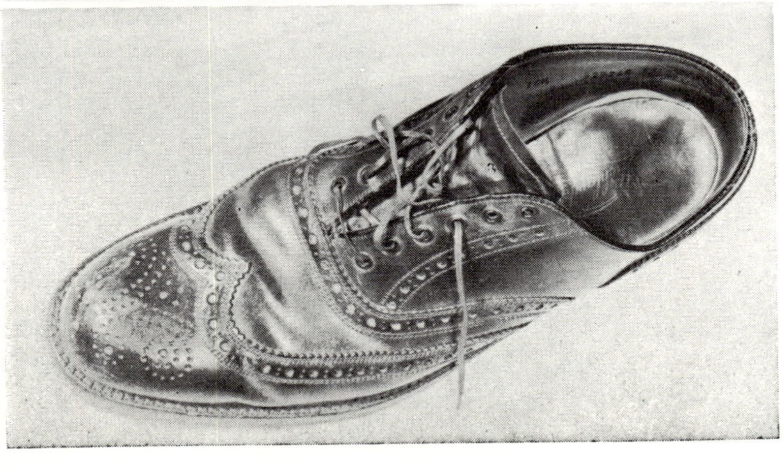

the shoe which creates discomfort for the patient. A heavy-duty shank should extend from midheel to just behind the heads of the metatarsals. The material used is 17-7 x .064 shaped and tempered stainless steel. The limited ankle joint brace requires a heavy-duty shank because the standard steel shank that is found, even in orthopedic shoes, is not strong enough to take the stress. Without the heavy-duty shank, the rivets holding the stirrup pull out, making the brace useless and ruining the shoe.

The shoe should be leather with a detachable heel and a stitched-on sole. The all leather shoe will last much longer than a paper-filled one. The shoe should have a Blucher opening with at least four eyelets. The Blucher-style shoe has two flaps that come off the vamp of the shoe and cover the instep of the foot, making a larger opening for the foot to enter the shoe (Fig. 6). When the shoe is laced and tied, the flaps covering the instep hold the foot much better than does the Balmoral-style shoe. The Balmoral has a small "V" type opening; it is more difficult for the foot to enter the shoe, and it cannot be laced as tightly (Fig. 6). The detachable heel makes it easier for the orthotist to attach the brace to the shoe and for the patient to keep good heels on his shoes.

SUMMARY

In summary, our experience indicates that a double adjustable ankle short-leg brace with a heavy-duty shank, with or without a dorsiflexion assist, and a good leather shoe is the brace of choice for the patient with hemiplegia.

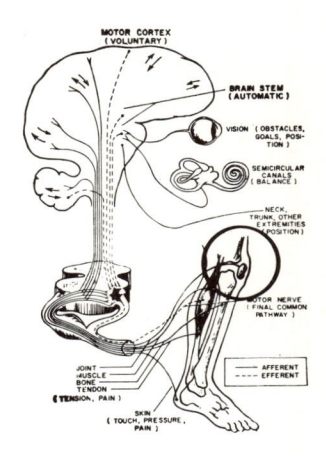

STRUCTURAL INSUFFICIENCY

I. Pathomechanics

JACQUELIN PERRY, M.D.

Structural sufficiency refers to the strength of the materials and the alignment of parts. The materials of concern to the physician and physical therapist are the bones and ligaments of the weight-bearing extremity. As is true of all other materials, they will yield to excessive strain. Yet, because they are viable structures, the stress stimulates reparative processes which add stability. At the same time, unfortunately, stress causes interference with joint function through formation of excessive fibrous tissue and osteophytes, and pain.

Joint utilization which avoids such strain and attempted repair, will prolong the patient's ability to walk. This prolongation of walking tolerance is represented both in the endurance for the immediate task as well as in the number of months and years of activity which will be possible.

Alignment determines the ease with which the joints are stabilized for effective weight bearing, the amount of shifting needed to balance the trunk over one limb, and the degree of stress on the ligaments and bones. Standing with normal joint alignment permits the body weight to be passed directly down the femur onto the vertical tibia and then onto the foot.

Muscular activity is needed only to balance the segments as they tend to lean one way and then the other. If the knee loses its ability to extend completely, the work of standing is increased in dramatic proportions, for now part of the body weight is behind the axis of the knee joint and the quadriceps muscles actually have to support that amount of weight (Fig. 1).

FORCES ON THE KNEE JOINT

For a qualitative relationship, the engineering staff at Rancho Los Amigos Hospital calculated the amount of force one might expect on a joint while a person is standing with his knee in different degrees of flexion (Fig. 2). With a 10-degree knee flexion contracture, the patellar pressure is 14 per cent of the body weight. This increases to 70 per cent of the body weight with a 20-degree contracture and to at least 140 per cent of body weight at a 30-degree position.

Because the total quadriceps mechanism consists of a fibrous sheath that encases three-fifths of the circumference of the knee, these pressures are also representative of the compressive

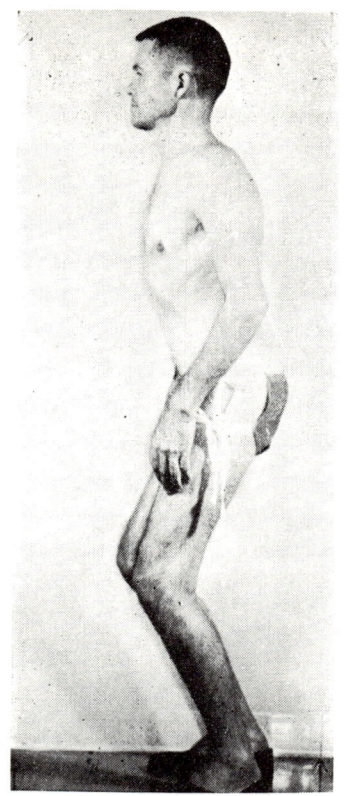

FIG. 1. Standing with knee flexion deformities demands much more work by the quadriceps as well as by the hip and ankle extensors.

JOINT TENSION WITH KNEE FLEXION

Knee Flexion	Joint Compression	
	P	J
10°	0.14BW	1.01BW
20°	0.70	1.20
30°	1.40	1.60
40°	2.40	2.60
50°	3.80	3.90
60°	5.30	5.40

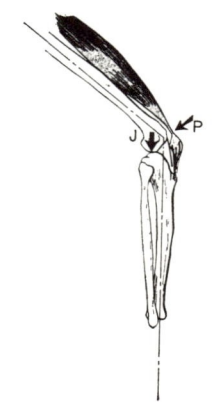

FIG. 2. The amount of compression expected at the patello-femoral junction (P) and at the tibia-femoral joint line (J) during standing in different degrees of knee flexion was calculated. The values are expressed in fractions of body weight (BW).

PATHOMECHANICS

force on the structures within the knee joint—a factor of great significance to the arthritic patient with his swollen, boggy joint lining.

Swelling and overgrowth of the synovial lining are reactions to injury. The insult may be the primary rheumatic process or it may be the result of the additional mechanical trauma of trying to perform in the face of disability. Therefore, walking with a significant degree of flexion contracture is not only painful, but is an aggravating factor in the disease process.

This has been reinforced clinically by Clayton's observation that his patients first demonstrate a significant disturbance in walking when they develop a flexion contracture of 20 degrees.[1] Few patients continue the struggle to walk when they approach a 45-degree flexion contracture.

The calculated patellar-femoral pressures are also representative of the work that the quadriceps must do to prevent the knee from collapsing on weight bearing. Thus the ability of a paretic patient to walk depends upon the balance between contracture and quadriceps strength, or upon his ability to substitute by leaning forward. This substitution posture requires strong hip and ankle extensor support. It becomes obvious that there is no such thing as a minor flexion contracture if any paralysis or joint pathology is present.

Knee Valgus Deformity

Knee valgus is restricted by tension of the medial collateral ligament and its extensions (Fig. 3). The lateral thrust that accompanies the shift of weight over the foot as single limb balance starts is a threat with each step (Fig. 4).

Normally, protection is offered by the overlying musculature. However, the patient with arthritis will avoid contracting these muscles as much as possible to escape the painful compressive force that such muscular tension would create in the knee joint. Thus, he unwittingly accepts unprotected lateral stress every time he bears weight (Fig. 5). This stress not only pulls on the medial supporting ligaments but also causes damaging compressive forces on the lateral condyles of the joint. The result is increasing erosion of the joint surfaces and actual compression of the supporting bones.

The bones of the arthritic have become softened by the hyperemia of inflammation, by relative inactivity and by palliative cortisone

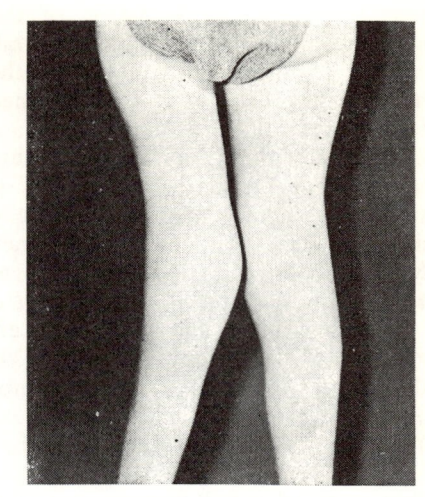

FIG. 3. This girl contracted poliomyelitis at one year of age, with most of the residual problem in the left lower extremity. She had Poor hip abductors, quadriceps and hamstrings. The foot muscles were adequate. The valgus deformity on the left reflects inadequate medial support of the knee and the exaggerated lateral trunk shift she used to substitute for inadequate hip abductor muscles.

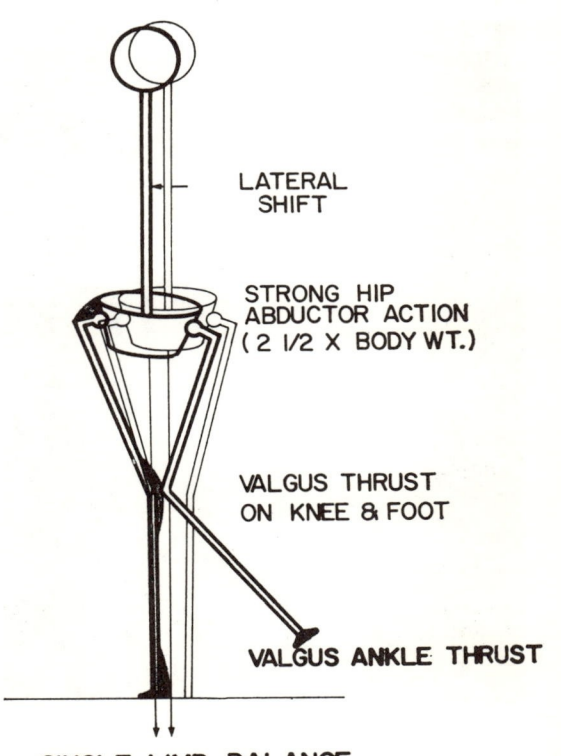

FIG. 4. In order to stand on one foot, a normal person shifts his trunk laterally about 1 inch while the leg and foot remain stationary. This creates a valgus thrust on the knee which normally is protected by the medial knee muscles.

therapy. Structural deformation of the tibia and the ligaments causes increasing valgus at the knee. The greater angulation of the knee joint magnifies the stress on the knee and, therefore, is a self-perpetuating mechanism to produce greater deformity and more disability.

Medial ligament laxity and valgus angulation of the tibia are common sequelae of paralysis following poliomyelitis contracted in early childhood (Fig. 3). The tibia actually grows crooked as a result of unequal stress on the epiphyseal plate and joint surfaces. The lateral side of the epiphyseal plate is discouraged from growing by the excessive compressive force, whereas the medial side is actually encouraged to grow by the relief of tension (Fig. 6).

The worst deformities are seen in those patients who have inadequate hip abductor musculature so that they exaggerate the lateral shift of the substituting mechanism for hip joint control upon weight bearing. The gluteus medius limp which is one cause of valgus deformity at the knee, is an example of this problem.

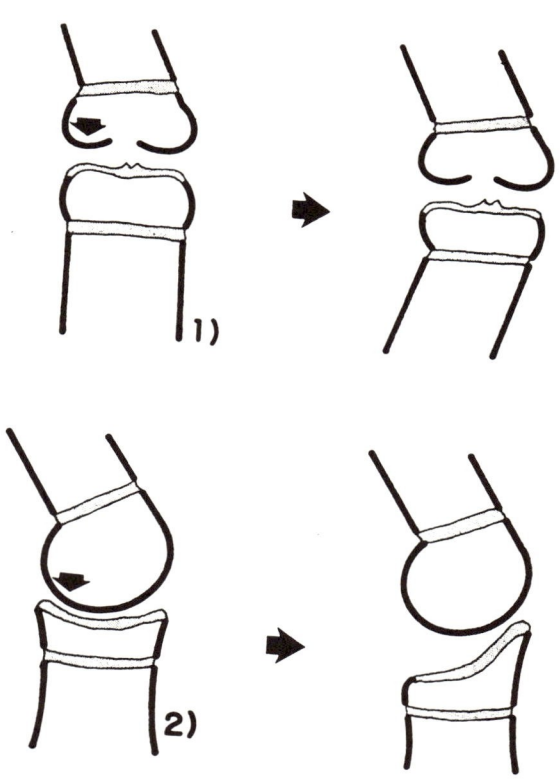

FIG. 6. Asymmetrical weight bearing stress causes permanent deformation of growing bone. There are two sites of action: (1) asymmetrical growth of the epiphyseal line and (2) unequal contouring of the joint surfaces.

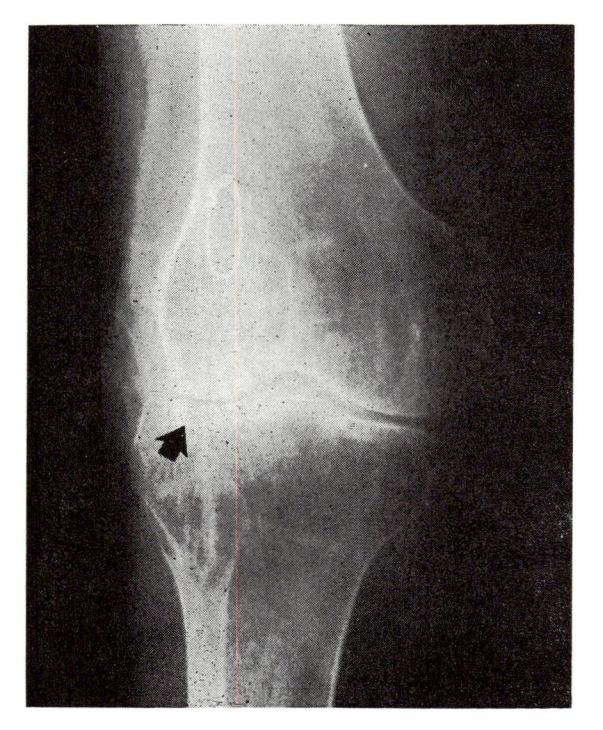

FIG. 5. Sclerosis of the adjacent articular margins of the lateral femoral and tibial condyles and narrowing of the joint space due to cartilage erosion, indicates a pathological response to concentrated stress. The unilateral nature of the joint pathology is evidence of the valgus thrust on weight bearing.

Recurvatum Deformity

The most marked ligamentous adaptation to strain is encouraged in the posterior capsule of the knee joint when a growing child substitutes hip and ankle extension for the absent quadriceps; or when he walks over an equinus contracture at the ankle. In order to stand erect, the body weight must be aligned over the forefoot. To accomplish this with the knee straight there must be 10 degrees of dorsiflexion available at the ankle. When the tibia is tipped backwards because strong calf activity is being used to prevent the knee from flexing, or because there is a fixed equinus contracture, the body weight pulls the femur for-

PATHOMECHANICS

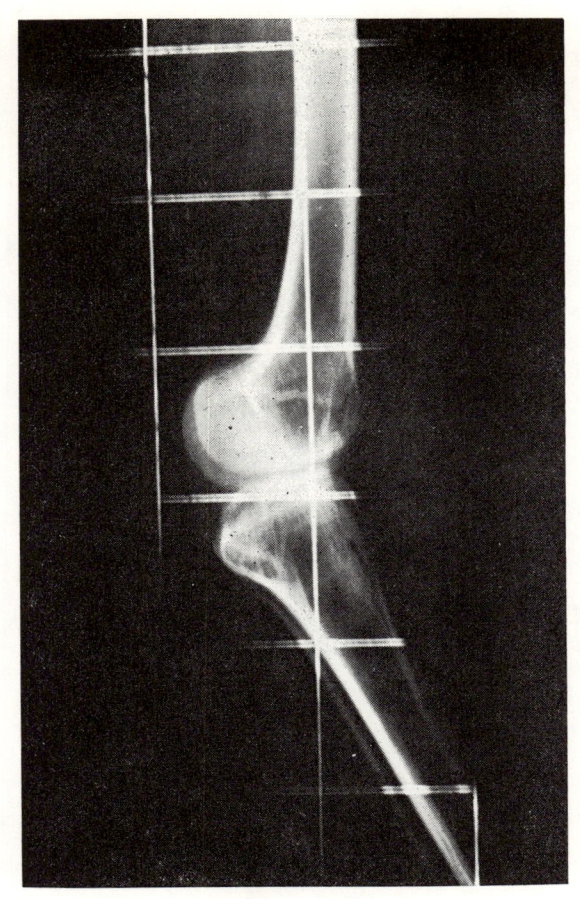

FIG. 7. This severe recurvatum of the knee is the result of massive overstretching of the posterior joint capsule and ligaments. The patient has Zero quadriceps, Poor hip extensors and an equinus contracture. The deformity developed because this child walked despite the equinus contracture. She must wear a long brace to avoid knee pain even though she could be brace-free if the deformity did not exist.

ward and there is a resulting hyperextension force on the knee joint (Fig. 7). With the added force of momentum during walking, this trend to recurvatum is exaggerated.

EFFECTS OF AGING

The adult will restrict his walking because of pain if the tissue stress becomes excessive. However, the ligaments of the young child yield so that there is progressive lengthening and a subsequent increasing laxity of the joint. Once again, the progressive malalignment exaggerates the deforming force and the cycle of a self-perpetuating mechanism for progressive deformation is begun. As the tissues lose their succulence and their ability to accommodate with aging, the joints become painful. Their management is now extremely difficult because of the tremendous mechanical disadvantages of deformed bones and lax ligaments. Adults who otherwise could have walked brace free had they been protected during their growing years, will be forced to use braces for stability. Experience demonstrates that it is inappropriate to plan on children getting along with the aid of postural stability, for this will lead to deleterious accommodations of the tissue and the encouragement of deformity. It is better to brace children, even to the point of excess, during their growing years so they then will have structural stability for the longer life span of adulthood.

REFERENCE

1. Clayton, Mack, Orthopaedic Surgeon, Denver, Colorado. Personal communication.

II. Structural Insufficiencies of the Knee in Rheumatoid Arthritis

VIRGINIA SCARAMUZZA GUESS, B.S.

RHEUMATOID ARTHRITIS is a chronic or recurrent inflammatory disorder characterized by involvement of any or all of the structures of the joint.

The initial symptoms of pain, joint swelling, and stiffness that occur early in the disease result from edema and inflammation of the joint capsule, a process which leads to thickening of the synovial membrane. The accumulation of fluid stretches the soft tissues around the joint and eventually the ligaments and the tendons are destroyed as a result of the excessive pressures. The cartilage erodes and the joint becomes lax and unstable.

As the muscles around the joint contract, the compression force on the edematous and inflamed tissue causes pain in the joint. As a result, the patient avoids using his muscles and atrophy eventually occurs. The joint is held in flexion which is the position that allows the greatest volume within the synovial cavity. In this position, the joint accommodates to the increase in fluid and gives the patient some relief of pain. If the joint continues to be held in this flexed position, contracture deformities occur.

THE KNEE JOINT

The knee is the most commonly involved joint which interferes with lower-extremity use. An unstable knee in rheumatoid arthritis results in pain, deformity, and loss of function. The goal of physical therapy is to provide support to the knee joint through muscular strengthening and the reduction or prevention of de-

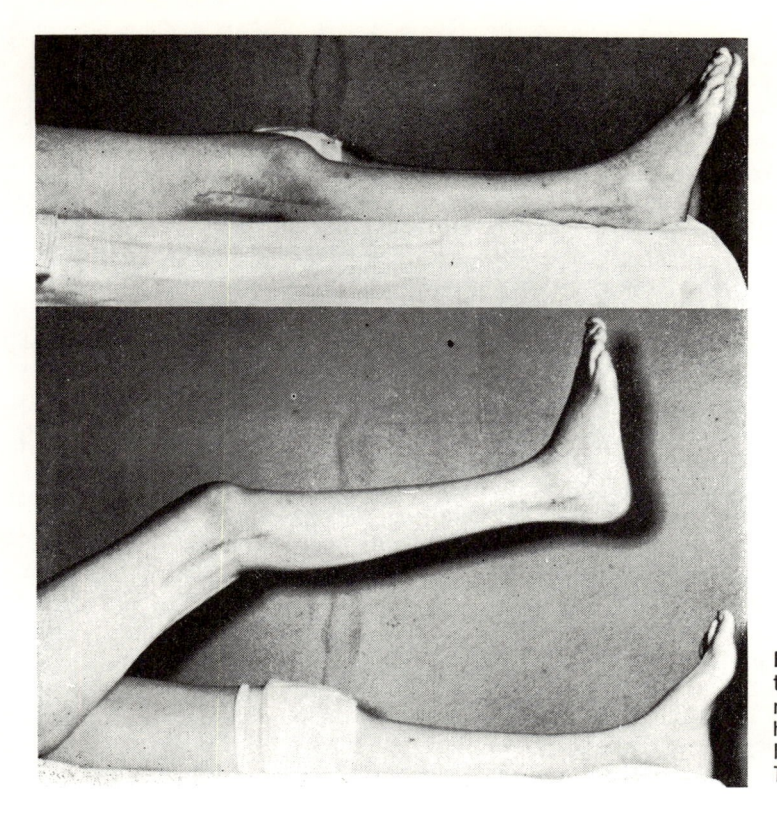

FIG. 1. This patient with rheumatoid arthritis evidences full passive knee extension range (top). However, he is not able to hold the knee in full extension on straight leg raising and it falls into flexion (below). The "lag" is 30 degrees in this case.

formity. To accomplish this goal, bracing for external support or surgery also may be necessary.

In evaluating the knee joint, three important problems must be identified: muscular weakness, the degree of flexion contracture, and ligamentous instability. An exercise and positioning program may provide adequate support for the knee if the deformity and ligamentous instability are not excessive. Bracing and surgery are used for correction when the problems are more severe.

Muscular Weakness

Contraction of the muscles around a joint filled with excessive fluid causes pain by further increasing the intra-articular pressure. To protect themselves from the pain, patients with arthritis tend to avoid using these muscles either for motion or support. As a result, the muscles weaken and further add to the ligamentous instability because the usual primary response to stress (*i.e.*, muscular contraction) has been avoided.

Disuse of the knee extensor muscles is a particularly serious problem in the arthritic knee because the fibrous expansion of the quadriceps encloses approximately three-fifths of the anterior surface of the knee. The patient loses medial and lateral as well as anterior support when this muscle group is inactive during periods of stress.

Inadequacy of the quadriceps to pull through full extension can be observed by comparing the difference between active and passive knee extension range, the difference being known as a "lag."

Such a "lag" of motion can be evaluated by asking the patient with rheumatoid arthritis to hold the knee in maximum extension and attempt to do straight leg raising. If the knee falls into any flexion as the extremity is raised, it is indicative that the patient lacks sufficient quadriceps strength to hold the knee in a full range of extension (Fig. 1), and hence is unable to give the knee the needed protection for safe weight bearing.

Strengthening. The goal of quadriceps strengthening is to increase strength sufficiently so that the joint can be supported adequately even if the ligaments have been destroyed. Muscular disuse around painful knee joints necessitates proper instruction of the patient in quadriceps "setting." Good isolated quadriceps contraction should be done fifty times per hour. When the patient learns control and awareness of the knee extensor muscles, progressive resistive exercise is important to obtain maximum strength. Either the isotonic or the isometric method can be used but must be approached with caution. If pain persists or increases one hour after exercise, an excessive amount of weight has been used. The weight should be decreased at the next treatment session. The isometric technique of strengthening is usually the method of choice for severely involved painful joints since muscular contraction is obtained without joint motion and the patient generally experiences less pain. Isometric exercise is done using a six-second hold.

Emphasis in the exercise program is placed on elimination of any "lag" of motion so that the active and the passive range of knee extension will be equal. If the patient has a lag of motion, a plaster resting splint is customarily used to support the knee joint during exercise. This permits straight leg raising to be done without stress on the knee joint (Fig. 2).

When the patient's strength increases, resistance can be added to straight leg raising while the knee continues to be supported by the splint.

"Hamstring" setting should not be neglected. Proper instruction in this exercise is important to gain knee flexion range following any immobilization of the knee. During the period of immobilization, alternate quadriceps and hamstring muscle setting exercises will provide some stability around the knee joint.

Knee Flexion Contracture

Deformity of the knee results in an imbalance of forces on the joint during weight bearing. Normally, the knee is most stable in full extension. Since knee flexion contractures are a common deformity, a proper positioning and plaster splinting program is important to gain full extension of the knee. The prone position, with the knees extended, must become a daily routine for patients with rheumatoid arthritis. An active program of splinting with plaster of Paris splints is used to correct knee flexion contractures. These splints can be made by the physical therapist and are used as an important adjunct to treatment. The knee is splinted in its range of maximum extension and is kept in this position except during exercise periods. The splints are changed every three to five days until a plateau in knee extension range is reached. When full knee extension is gained, the splint is worn only at night to prevent the flexion contracture from recurring.

Corrective splinting to reduce knee flexion contracture is effective as long as the tibia moves forward on the femur. The physical therapist must be alert to the danger of pos-

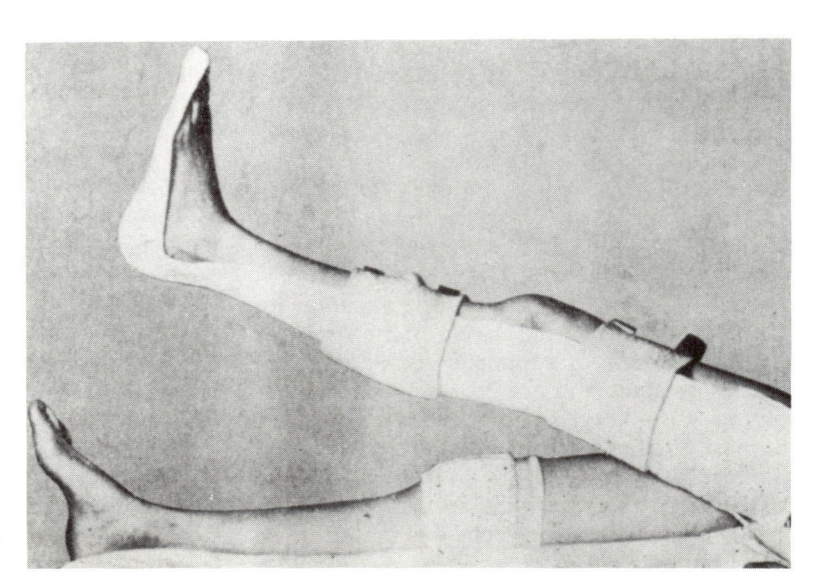

FIG. 2. A posterior resting splint protects the knee during straight leg raising. The splint on this patient is the final stage of a sequential splinting program to reduce a knee flexion deformity.

terior subluxation and determine if it is present when the splints are changed. If subluxation is suspected, further corrective splinting is discontinued and a splint is used only to maintain the correction already gained. A surgical procedure may be necessary before further improvement in extension can be made.

Limited Flexion Range. Occasionally, following a knee synovectomy, loss of range of motion in flexion occurs. This is common in arthritic children who are unable to exercise through even minimal pain. In these children, an anterior flexion splint is indicated (Fig. 3). Such a splint is used to maintain and increase the range of knee flexion. The extension and the flexion splints must be used alternately in order to maintain the full range of knee extension while gaining flexion. When an anterior flexion splint is used, the physical therapist must assume the responsibility to make sure that knee flexion contractures do not occur. Knee extension is the stable position. Extension range must not be sacrificed for flexion range. With the physical therapist's close observation and planning of the time that each splint is worn, the patient will maintain extension as he increases flexion.

Ligamentous Instability

The third problem in the patient with an arthritic knee is ligamentous instability. Strong knee extensors in a knee free of deformity can compensate for ligamentous instability and can adequately support the knee joint even if the ligaments are destroyed. However, when quadriceps strengthening and the attainment of full knee extension are not adequate to provide knee stability, a brace can provide external stability for the knee joint. A knee cage with an anterior control, a long-leg brace with a pretibial shell, or a conventional long-leg brace are available means of gaining external stability. The selection of the type of brace depends on the individual needs of the patient. When a brace is being considered, the ability of the patient to put on and take off the brace by himself should be considered. A patient who cannot handle the brace by himself may resist wearing such a device.

The Knee Cage. A knee cage is a temporary brace which has medial and lateral bars that extend upward on the thigh and down to the ankle joint (Fig. 4). It has posterior thigh and calf cuffs and an anterior knee control. To encourage knee extension, the lateral supports must extend from just below the gluteal fold to just above the malleoli of the ankle. Short lateral bars which reach only to midthigh and midcalf, actually encourage rather than prevent flexion. The knee cage is effective as an assistive support for the quadriceps in patients who have a "lag" of motion

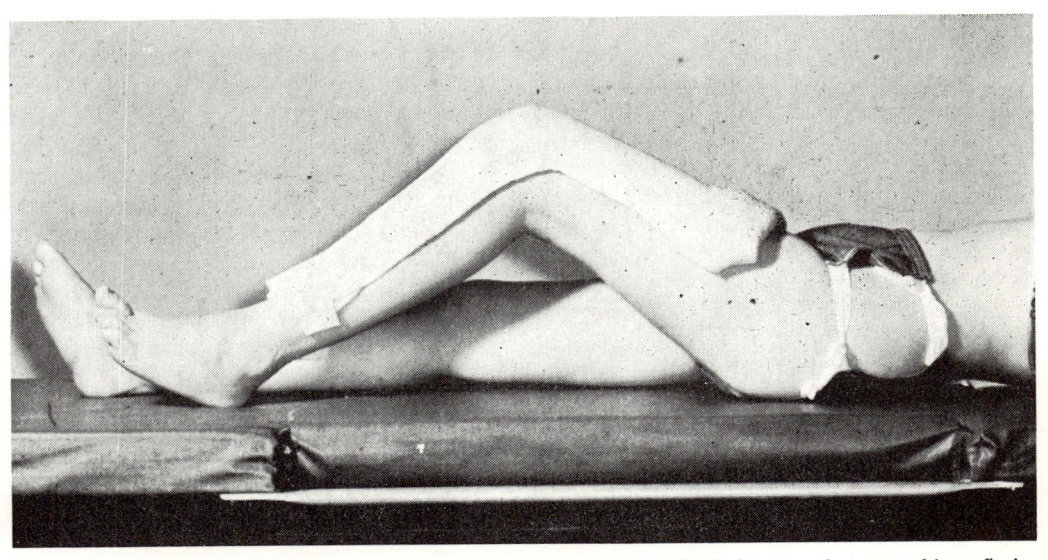

FIG. 3. The anterior resting splint is used alternately with a posterior splint to increase the range of knee flexion (commonly postoperatively) while maintaining extension range.

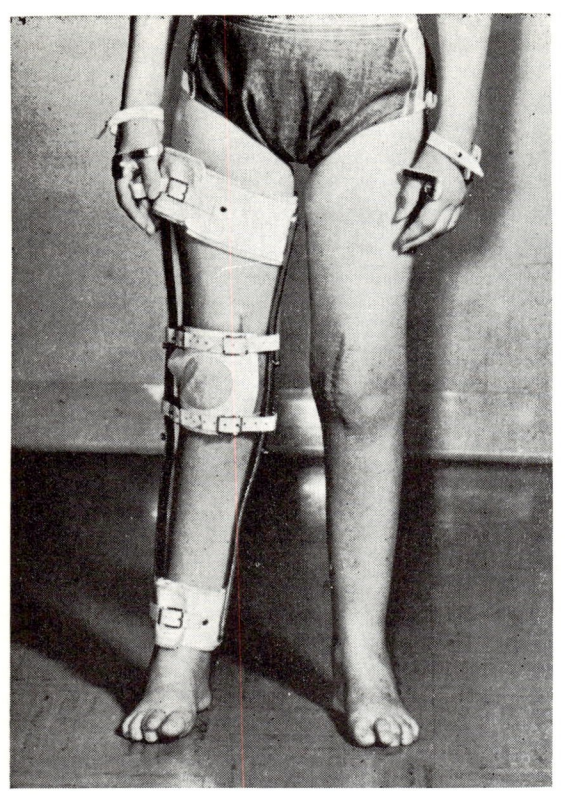

FIG. 4. The knee cage. To encourage knee extension, the lateral and medial bars should extend from as high as possible on the thigh to just above the ankle. Shorter bars which reach from midthigh to midcalf actually encourage flexion rather than correcting it.

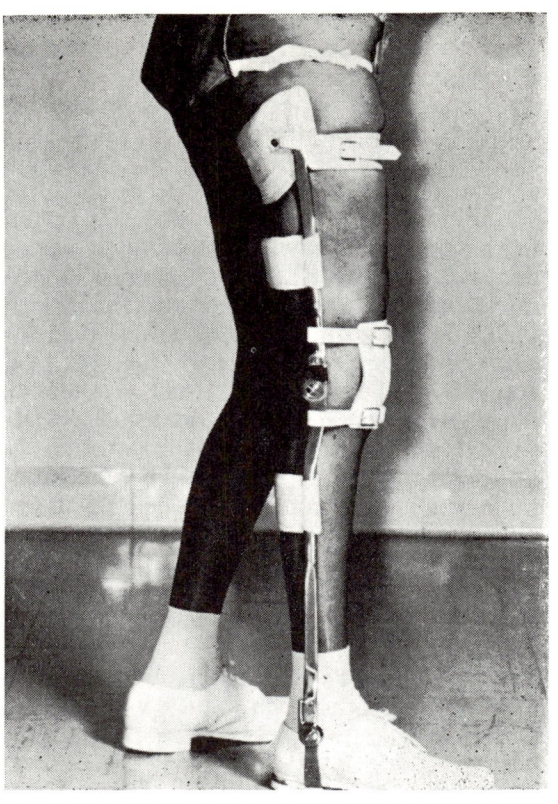

FIG. 5. The standard long-leg brace used for weight-bearing on a severely involved joint.

between active and passive knee extension. Also, it offers assistance to the quadriceps on weight bearing. The support is worn until the increase in quadriceps strength makes the passive and the active range of motion equal. By fastening the anterior knee control loosely, the quadriceps are allowed to continue to contract during walking. The control is used as an assist when applied in this manner. This type of knee cage can be easily removed and the patient may be allowed to walk without support for short periods of time—until the knee extensor muscles demonstrate signs of fatigue.

Another effective use of the knee cage is for a postoperative knee, or for a quadriceps that has been overstretched as the result of a prolonged knee flexion contracture. The knee cage can be used temporarily until the quadriceps adapts to its new length.

The Long-Leg Brace. Occasionally, a conventional long-leg brace is used to give the patient support for weight bearing on a severely involved knee joint (Fig. 5). The long-leg brace holds the knee in the stable extended position. The uprights and the anterior knee control of the brace provide support to the entire extremity.

This added support decreases the amount of force applied to the knee joint, and thus may indirectly decrease knee pain on weight bearing.

The Pretibial Shell. The most successful permanent brace for unstable knee deformities in our experience is a long-leg brace with a pretibial shell (Fig. 6). The pretibial shell is particularly effective against a valgus deformity.

It provides proper alignment of the knee and distributes the stabilizing forces over a

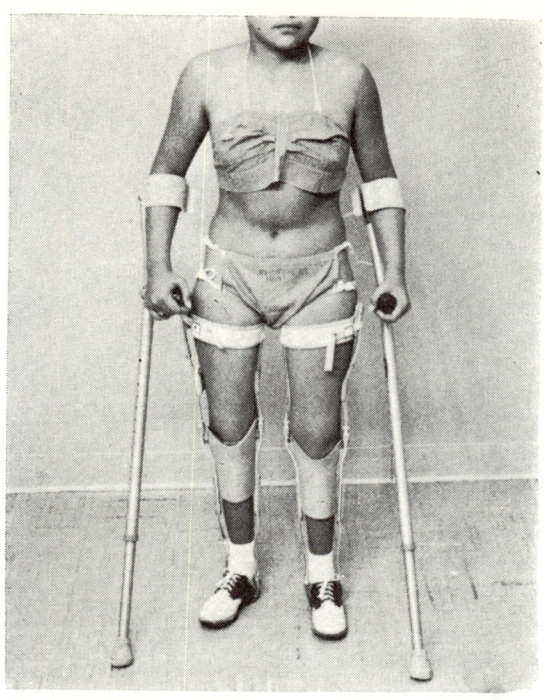

FIG. 6. The long-leg brace with pretibial shell. The addition of the shell provides proper alignment of the knee and distributes the stabilizing forces over a wide area.

large area. Ligaments and muscles are unable to control a valgus deformity in an arthritic knee when it is the result of bony deterioration. As the deformity increases, more pain and stress occur at the knee joint during ambulation. In time, the increased pain will limit walking if the deformity is not controlled.

SUMMARY

Lack of activity is devastating to a patient with rheumatoid arthritis. Swollen, painful knee joints should not be an indication for complete bedrest. Such inactivity will result in greater loss of functional ability. Muscular strength must be maintained even during periods of exacerbation of the disease. The exercise program often needs modification according to the patient's activity tolerance, but muscle "setting" and isometric exercise which can retard loss of strength are still possible. The goal in treating the unstable knee of the patient with rheumatoid arthritis is to provide stability by muscular strengthening and reduction of deformity.

Bracing can contribute to this goal as an assistive device during an intensive quadriceps strengthening program. It is also a means of producing support for the knee that is too severely damaged to rely on muscular strengthening alone.

At times, a combination of surgery and bracing are needed to accomplish the final goal of a stable knee joint on weight bearing.

III. Bracing Design for Knee Joint Instability

DAVID HEIZER, C.O.

Supporting or applying corrective forces to the deformed knee poses a difficult orthotic program. To be effective, the mechanical design of the long-leg brace requires correcting and stabilizing forces to be of large magnitude. Yet, there is a limit posed by the pressure tolerance of the skin and deeper tissues overlying the bony prominences.

The standard condyle pad used with long leg braces confines the forces to a small area (Fig. 1). If there is severe deformity, the pressure required to correct it is usually beyond the patient's tolerance. As a result, the common procedure is to repeatedly adjust the brace to accommodate to the patient's deformity as it gradually gets worse.

To overcome this difficulty, a molded pretibial shell has been substituted for condyle pads during the past four years (Fig. 1). It offers better control of the knee, more comfort, and less skin irritation by spreading the corrective pressures at the knee over a much larger area. The pretibial shell has been used to provide stability or to gain correction in patients with valgus, varus, flexion or recurvatum deformities of the knee. The clinical conditions treated have been poliomyelitis, arthritis, spinal cord injury, cerebral palsy and Charcot-joint pathology. Regular use of the orthosis by the growing child will provide some permanent correction of the deformity, particularly knee flexion or valgus. We have not seen any structural change in a patient who has full growth. The pretibial shell has made it possible to improve alignment, hence better brace tolerance and more stable walking can be gained in patients of all ages.

The relative effectiveness of the two methods can be compared by looking at the forces required (Fig. 2). The force against the knee needed to support 5 degrees of valgus in a 100-pound person would be about 9 pounds.

BRACE DESIGN FOR STRUCTURAL INSTABILITY

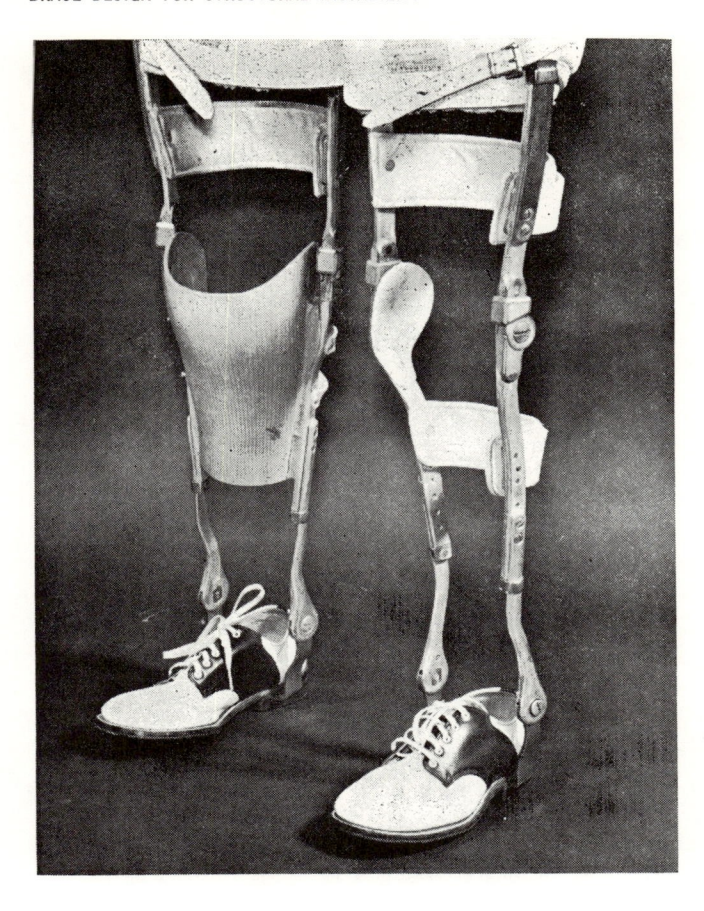

FIG. 1. The standard medial support for the knee is a condyle pad as shown on the brace at the right. This concentrates the supporting force in a small area. A pretibial shell (left) provides more comfort and better support because the force is dispersed over a larger area.

If this same patient had 25 degrees of valgus, the force requirement would increase to about 47 pounds. A well-shaped condyle pad covers about 4 square inches. This would place about 12 pounds of force per square inch against the medial condyle of the knee. Unfortunately, many pads are not well-shaped. They are too flat and cause spot pressure on the bony prominence of the femoral condyle. In these instances the pressure may be increased to 20 or 30 pounds. The molded plastic pretibial shell covers about 29 square inches and in the above example would reduce the medial condyle pressure to about 1.5 pounds per square inch to correct the same degree of valgus.

Three points of pressure are needed to correct any deformity, and the same is true at the knee (Fig. 3). When utilizing a long-leg brace, the three points are the thigh band, a knee support (in this case the pretibial shell), and the shoe. In the case of valgus, the thigh band provides a lateral force, the knee pressure is medial, and at the shoe the force is lateral.

The height of the thigh band is dictated by the type of deformity being treated and hence the amount of leverage necessary. Shoe requirements are dictated by the type of ankle joint needed. In turn, the type of ankle joint selected is determined by the amount of muscular control present; the joint may be free, limited, or locked.

The pretibial shell is constructed from a cast of the patient's knee. At the time the orthotist makes the tracing and the cast, he holds the extremity in the position of maximum correction. A washed stockinette is put on the leg and bony prominences outlined with an indelible pencil. The plaster bandage is applied and carefully molded to the leg to insure an intimate fit of the shell. The indelible makings on the stockinette are transferred from the negative mold when a postive mold is made. The knee is also checked for lateral instability as this information indicates the amount of support needed and the way the shell should be cut.

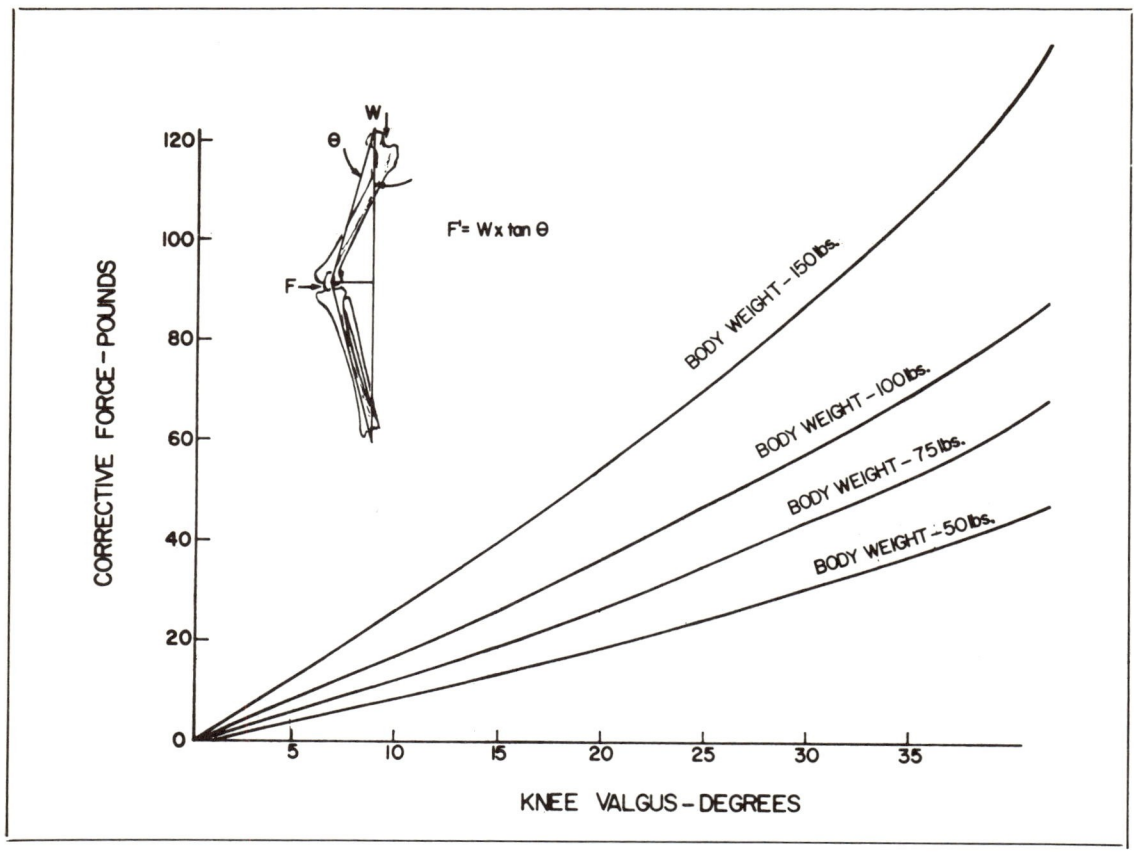

FIG. 2. Illustrates the amount of force required to correct varying degrees of knee valgus deformity in patients with different body weights.

VALGUS DEFORMITY

The orthotist tries to get as much correction as possible when he makes the tracing and cast prior to fabricating the brace. By holding the knee in about 5 degrees of flexion, he can usually obtain complete correction of the valgus condition, though his success depends upon the laxity of the lateral ligaments and the severity of the deformity. Occasionally, the orthotist can obtain only a percentage of correction at the first casting. After the patient has worn the brace for a time, additional correction may be obtained. If valgus is the only knee deformity, the pretibial shell will be cut so that the medial side is high enough to cover the medial condyle of the femur while the lateral side will be cut off below the lateral condyle (Fig. 3). This assures corrective force where it is needed and prevents obstructive counter forces. However, if there is ligamentous instability laterally, the shell is trimmed so that it covers both the medial and lateral condyles of the femur to give good support to the knee. The thigh band is shaped so that it reaches the greater trochanter. This gives a long lever and a solid point of fixation.

KNEE FLEXION DEFORMITY

In treating knee flexion contractures, the techniques of construction are the same with the exception that the alignment efforts are directed toward straightening the knee flexion contracture. The pretibial shell is trimmed high both medially and laterally so that the condyles are covered and good support is given to the knee. To make the brace wearable, the residual flexion of the knee must be incor-

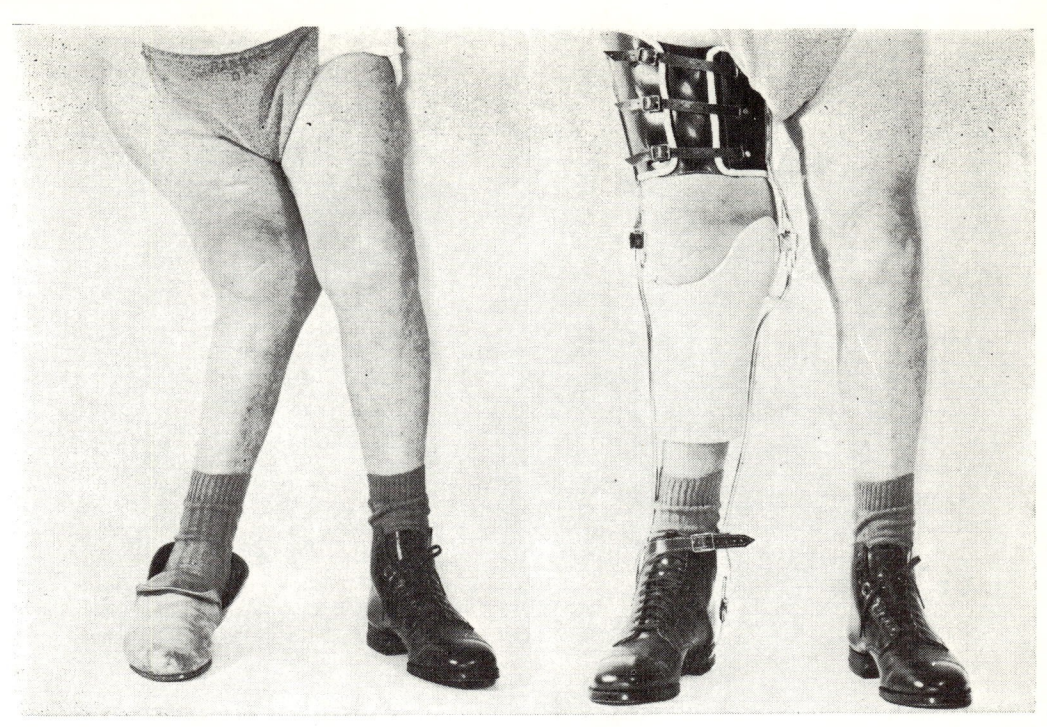

FIG. 3. This patient has a Charcot-knee joint secondary to lumbo-sacral root damage. He had ceased to walk because of the severity of his valgus deformity (left). A long-leg brace with a pretibial shell having a high medial flange (right) provided the necessary stability for safe ambulation.

porated in the brace. This can be accomplished by the use of a fan-lock (Fig. 4), a dial-lock (Fig. 5), or by flexing the brace bars.

When the patient needs to walk with a locked-knee joint, the fan-lock is indicated as it allows the knee joint to be locked in different degrees of extension. The unit (made of .060 stainless steel) has a series of adjustment holes approximately $7/32$-inch apart. This permits about 5 degrees difference in joint position with each interval.

The dial-lock is desirable when the patient is able to walk with a free knee but needs accommodation to a fixed flexion deformity. Being constructed with a long curved slot, motion is restricted in one direction according to the placement of the locking screw while allowing free travel along the rest of the arc. Thus the brace can be set to restrict either flexion or extension but allows free motion in the other direction.

The third means of accommodating to a knee flexion contracture is by flexing the brace bars distal to the knee joint. This method is the least effective because it weakens the brace bars, subjecting them to breakage, and it allows no means for adjustment as the patient improves. The thigh band does not need to be particularly high as the absence of lateral thrust negates the need to gain fixation from the trochanter.

RECURVATUM DEFORMITY

When bracing for recurvatum, the knee is placed in slight flexion and again the pretibial shell is trimmed high on both the medial and lateral sides of the knee.

The midthigh band is set lower than usual to help keep the knee in flexion. A 90-degree downstop is put in the ankle joint with a dorsiflexion assist if needed. The thigh band need not be high on the lateral side since there is no tendency for valgus when the knee is in flexion. A posterior strap is added to the pretibial shell to keep the leg in contact with the shell. Otherwise, the leg might move forward and back during ambulation causing discomfort and skin breakdown.

As illustrated by the patient with a Charcot-knee deformity of about 35 degrees of valgus (Fig. 3), the severity of the deformity also

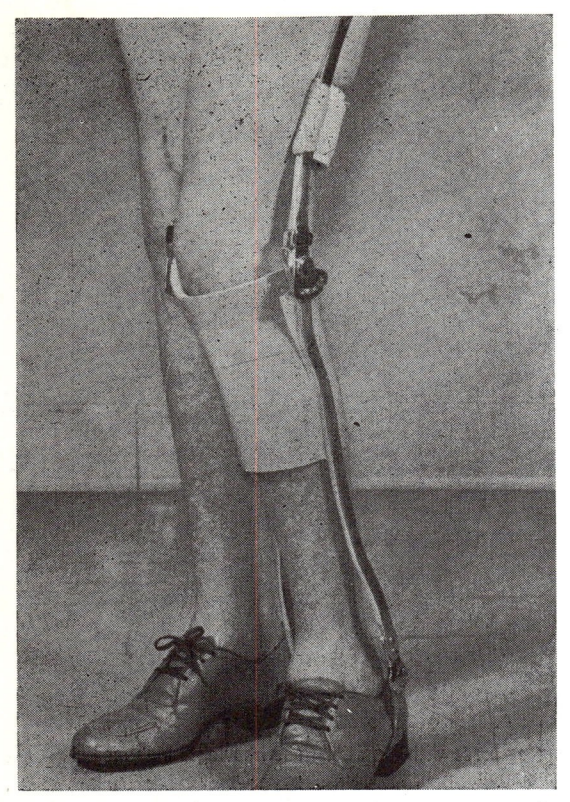

FIG. 4. A fan-lock at the knee permits the brace to be aligned in selective degrees of flexion.

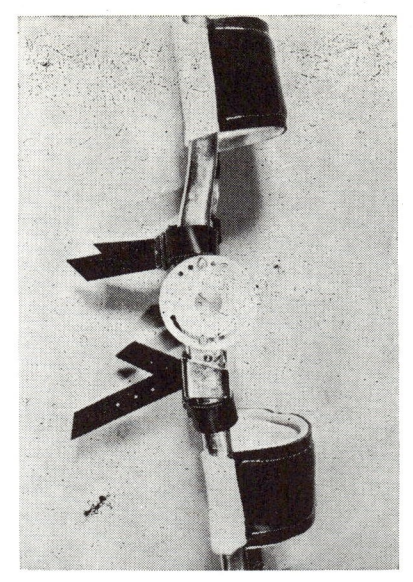

FIG. 5. The dial lock may be set to restrict either flexion or extension but it permits free motion in the other direction.

dictates the choice of materials to be used in the brace construction. The bars have to be strong enough to withstand the forces that will be put upon them. Therefore, $\frac{3}{4}$- x $\frac{3}{16}$-inch aluminum was chosen. Aluminum (0.090) was used for the thigh and midthigh bands to add sufficient strength to the brace. A lighter material would have allowed the brace to move, causing the bands to break or the rivets to shear off.

In contrast, lightness of the brace is emphasized when treating patients with rheumatoid arthritis because of the dominance of pain and skin sensitivity. The smallest size adult brace bar available from a commercial manufacturer is $\frac{5}{8}$ x $\frac{3}{16}$ inches. This is adequate for correcting most of the knee deformities in rheumatoid arthritis patients. Band stock of .090 thickness is used to add stability to the brace.

SUMMARY

It is our conclusion that the most effective way to control structural instability of the knee with a long-leg brace is to incorporate a pretibial shell to provide the necessary supportive or corrective forces at the knee without exceeding the patient's tolerance.

$5.00/2M/5880/1-81